PEOPLE ARE TALKING ABOUT LEAN FOR LIFE!

"I was self-conscious, fat, and fed up. I vowed to myself that I would do the program 100%—and I did. In five months, I lost more than 40 pounds!"

— *Margaret Kelman, 47*
Lost 50 pounds

"I lost 100 pounds in just ten months. My greatest thrill was hearing my seven-year-old granddaughter say, 'Gee, Grandma, now I can put my arms all the way around you.'"

— *June M. Griesemer, 69*
Lost 115 pounds

"Lean for Life is the only program I've ever tried where I didn't feel hungry."

— *John Morgan, 43*
Lost 63 pounds

"I'm an orchestra conductor, and the compliments and congratulations I've gotten since losing 90 pounds are music to my ears. But more important than how I look is how I feel—I have more energy than ever!"

— *Elizabeth Wright, 23*
Lost 90 pounds

"Before I became Lean for Life, I was too slow to try out for sports. But the program helped me lose weight, learn to eat right, build up my confidence, and get me in shape for football."

— *Eric Eastman, 13*
Lost 45 pounds

"This phenomenal program has given me back my life! I'm so grateful I found it."

— *Susan Gardanier, 37*
Lost 85 pounds

"I'm a baker and I love to eat, but I realized things had to change the day I tipped the scales at 299 pounds. I lost 106 pounds in eight months—and feel better than I ever have."

— *Vince Pilato, 36*
Lost 106 pounds

"The principles I've learned on the program have instilled a sense of discipline and focus—not only in the way I eat, but in my business life as well. Once I made up my mind to go for it, the process was painless."

— *Tim Klein, 49*
Lost 77 pounds

"I think different, I act different, and I look different. Lean for Life has changed my life. It works!"

— *Princess Leali, 34*
Lost 100 pounds

Lean
for
Life®

Lean for Life ®

The Clinically Proven Step-by-Step Plan for Losing Weight Rapidly and Safely... and Controlling It for Life!

Cynthia Stamper Graff

with Jerry Holderman

Foreword by

Peter Vash, M.D., M.P.H.

Assistant Clinical Professor, UCLA School of Medicine
Past President, American Society of Bariatric Physicians
Executive Medical Director, Lindora Medical Clinics

GRIFFIN PUBLISHING COMPANY

LIBRARY OF CONGRESS CATALOGING-IN-PUBLICATION DATA

Stamper Graff, Cynthia.
Lean for Life: The Clinically Proven Step-by-Step Plan for
Losing Weight Rapidly and Safely...and Controlling It
for Life! / by Cynthia Stamper Graff with Jerry Holderman.

1. Diet. 2. Weight Loss. 3. Health. 4. Fitness.
5. Nutrition. I. Jerry Holderman. II. Title.

ISBN 1-882180-63-1

Second Edition
Printed in the United States of America

10 9 8 7

Lean for Life® and Mitochondriac® are registered trademarks
of Lindora, Inc., Costa Mesa, California. BioModifier™,
BioModification™, BioMod™, and Mr. Mito™ are trademarked by
Lindora, Inc. MENTORS™ is the trademark for the Daily Mental Training
materials and program developed and owned by
Portland Health Institute, Inc., 1515 SW Fifth Ave., Suite 1021,
Portland, Oregon 97201. Used with permission.

This book is in no way intended to be a substitute for the medical advice of a personal physician. We advise and encourage the reader to consult his/her physician before beginning this or any other weight management and/or exercise program. The authors and the publisher disclaim any liability or loss, personal or otherwise, resulting from the procedures in this book.

An important part of any effort to improve your health is the decision to seek and use help from trusted health professionals from the very start. MENTORS Daily Mental Training is not intended as a substitute for such help, and the authors and manufacturers of MENTORS Daily Mental Training materials and programs disclaim all liability for any injury or illness sustained in connection with their use.

To my parents,

Marshall and Nell Stamper

"If you always do what you've always done,
you'll always get what you always got."

ANNE KAISER STEARNS

TABLE OF CONTENTS

Chapter 6

WEIGHT LOSS: WEEK 4   169

Day 22: The Power of Practice • Exercising Your Options: Making Fitness Fun • The Hidden Payoffs of Being Fat • Day 23: A Healthy Investment • Your Recipe for a Healthy, Satisfying Life • Day 24: Success Strategies for Meeting Real Life Challenges • How to Read Food Labels • Marketing 101: Food Shopping Made Easy • Day 25: Taking the Offensive: Overcoming Other "Real Life" Challenges • Have It Your Way: Healthy Choices in Restaurants • Now You're Cooking • The Morning Rush • Under the Weather? • Eating on the Job • Day 26: Go With the "Flow" • The Exhilaration of Exercise • Day 27: Preparing for "Phase 2: Metabolic Adjustment" • The Benefits • Day 28: The Past is a Present as You Proceed to the Future • What You've Learned • Measure Up

Chapter 7

"PHASE 2: METABOLIC ADJUSTMENT"   205

The 3 Levels of Metabolic Adjustment • How It Works and Why It's Essential • 12 Ways to Guarantee Results During Metabolic Adjustment

Chapter 8

"PHASE 3: LIFETIME MAINTENANCE"   229

The Challenge • Stabilizing at Your New Lean Weight • Achieving Equilibrium • Lean Foods vs. Fat Foods • "So What Do I Eat?" • "How Much Do I Eat?" • 10 Ways to Guarantee Results During Lifetime Maintenance • The Four Habits of Highly Successful Maintainers • The More You Listen, the More You Lose • What Stress Can Do to Your Body and Your Brain

ACKNOWLEDGMENTS

Cynthia Stamper Graff

This book wouldn't exist if it weren't for two very special families—the Stamper family and the Lindora family. I am blessed to be a member of both.

My father and mother, Marshall and Nell Stamper, are also the parents of Lindora. They raised both of us on the fundamental principles of positive expectation. I will always be grateful to them for believing in me and trusting that I could and would make appropriate "life choices." I am honored to share with others some of the wisdom I have learned from them.

I also thank my daughter, Ali, who always understood that while "Mommy's book" was very important, it was never more important than she is. I look forward to taking more trips to the park just as much as she does.

The loving support of my brothers, Steve Stamper and Bernie Stamper, my sister, Kitty Nordstrom, and their families also means a great deal to me. I appreciate their bearing with me during the writing of this book, especially when I seemed "preoccupied" at family functions.

The Lindora family has been equally supportive. Special thanks to:

Peter Vash, M.D., M.P.H., who was always accessible and wise with his input. Our Friday brainstorming sessions are consistently a highlight of my week, and the ideas generated during those working lunches continue to improve the program in very significant ways.

Jan Hunter, R.N., Director of Nursing, who with 17 years of experience with the Lindora program is truly a treasured resource. She possesses an intuitive grasp of the challenges our patients face in their struggles to lose weight, and her experience—both personal and professional—continues to enrich the program in countless ways.

Debbie Riley, L.V.N., Lindora's Nurse Educator, who has been tireless in her efforts to ensure that this book addressed the everyday problems our patients encounter. She is a vital and valued member of Lindora's "4:00A.M. Club," a group so psychically "in tune" that we often have the same idea at the same time—a fact that only becomes apparent when we read our E-mail and find that it jibes with our "brain mail."

Joe Risser, M.D., M.P.H., who has proven to be a fabulous addition to Team Lindora. He is a sensitive, caring physician who also happens to be a techno-wizard. I can always count on his thorough research and thoughtful analysis, and I appreciate both very much.

Olivia Moreno, my assistant and friend, who has been a real lifesaver more nights and weekends than either of us probably cares to remember. Thank you, Olivia!

Thank you, as well, to Ted Buetow, M.D., Andral Dugger, M.D., John Dubois, M.D., Lynn Nieto, N.P., and Cay Taylor, N.P., for their service to Lindora and the care they consistently show our patients, as well to Jackie Martinez, L.V.N., Terry Chronister, L.V.N., Vickie Flatt, L.V.N., Patti Sewell, L.V.N., Ryan Mariden, and Sherrie Theckston, for their ongoing efforts to help improve the Lindora program and the people who administer it.

Kathy Walker, R.N., Carol Mulvey, L.V.N., and Team Orange inspired the original "At Home" patients to make the lifestyle changes necessary for achieving lasting weight control. Their successful approach in reaching out to people unable to visit our clinics demonstrated that the principles of our program can truly work for anyone, anywhere.

I also appreciate Keith McGuinness, Rick Bullock, Mike Brkich , Mari Markell, Sausha Sherbin, Leonard Wright, Joanie Schreck, Melody Lucero, Pam Withers, and every member of Lindora's corporate team, whose commitment to helping people become Lean for Life was apparent every time they pulled together to support me when it seemed like I had three full-time jobs.

Team Lindora is comprised of the hundreds of women and men whose commitment to promoting good health and longevity makes a difference in the lives of many people every day. Without each of them, this book would not be what it is. They not only encouraged me with cards and calls, but encouraged their patients to share their stories so that others could benefit from their experiences. Special thanks to Cathy Markuson, L.V.N., Carol Kellum, L.V.N., Janise Pratt, Lisa Burden, L.V.N., Jayme Davidson, R.N., Carol Landis, L.V.N., Alisa Blansett, R.N., Maryanne Billings, Laura Rider, Audrey Smith, L.V.N., Pauline Garcia, L.V.N., Heather Ferber, Sue Slim, Carla Carney, and Deena Eshom, L.V.N.

Dr. Fred Saba's excellent work on creating and refining the Lean for Life web site is also very much appreciated. His expertise in the field of distance learning will make it possible to reach so many people. Eric Flamholtz and Yvonne Randle at Management Systems have helped Lindora become a stronger organization. The business disciplines they've helped us develop have strengthened the organization; this book is a result of the strategic planning we did together.

To my fellow YPO'ers, I thank you all—especially the members of my forum (you know who you are!). I constantly learn from each of you and from the "resources" available to us.

There are several people whose contributions in the field of obesity research have been especially meaningful to me. Thank you to George Blackburn, M.D., for the always outstanding Harvard Obesity Conferences. Every one has proven valuable in helping us further refine our program, and Dr. Blackburn's words of encouragement many years ago contributed to Lindora's strong commitment to research and data collection. Steven Phinney, M.D., Ph.D., and Dennis Jones, Ph.D. have conducted significant research that validates the efficacy and safety of ketosis in the dieting state; Tom Wadden, Ph.D., professor of psychology at the University of Pennsylvania School of Medicine, has provided encouragement and positive feedback about our program and has motivated me personally with his wonderful lectures on behavior modification and the importance of ongoing maintenance.

I want to acknowledge and thank Steven Blair, P.E.D., especially for his 1992 Harvard Conference lecture on the efficacy of exercising more often for shorter periods, which helped inspire Lindora's emphasis on movement and gentle exercise. Arturo Rolla, M.D. and his research also have been an inspiration. Richard Atkinson, M.D. deserves recognition for his vision in launching the American Obesity Association (AOA) and for his commitment to the compassionate clinical treatment of obesity. The research legacy of George Bray, M.D. has inspired Lindora to strive for continued improvement in providing unparalled patient care. And a very special thanks to John Foreyt, Ph.D., at Baylor University. His lectures on behavior modification are always enlightening, and I've found the dinners with him afterward particularly stimulating. I truly appreciate his belief in me and his encouragement of this project.

There are two professional organizations that have been enormously important to me personally, as well as to the development of the Lindora program. The research conducted by members of the North American Association for the Study of Obesity (NAASO) affords Lindora an opportunity to continue being "cutting edge." The American Society of Bariatric Physicians (ASBP) is dedicated to the principles of advancing ethical clinical treatment of the obese patient. Lindora has grown as an organization from the opportunities that ASBP has given us to share our experiences and to learn from other members.

I'm so happy to be collaborating with Harry Wexler, Ph.D., Ellen McGrath, Ph.D., Carol Lindquist, Ph.D., and their colleagues at the Psychology Center in Laguna Beach, California on an extraordinary project involving groundbreaking psychological testing of the overweight and obese. Our association gave me the added momentum to make this book even better when I was convinced I'd given it all I could.

Robert Schwartz listened to me talk "content" for hours and was always generous with ideas and material. Heartfelt thanks to Gloria Duboise, whose encouraging cards and notes seemed to always arrive at just the right time, and

Estelle Kevitch, a true friend who was always there. I also want to acknowledge Margaret Blackburn, who has been "another mother" to Ali and me. We both appreciate her very much. And to Karen Mabre—you said I could do it!

Roger Riddell deserves special thanks and a great big hug for encouraging me throughout the year this project required from start to finish. He once told me that a book is like a movie in that it's never "finished"—you just run out of time and money. From him, I learned to "let it go."

To Maury Povich and producer Liz Frillizia, my deepest appreciation. This book is, in large part, the result of the intense interest generated in the Lindora program by Diana Rosenfeld's numerous appearances on their show. I also appreciate the sensitivity that Kathleen Sullivan and the staff at Lifetime displayed while sharing Diana's story. And, of course, my deepest appreciation goes to Diana Rosenfeld and Tommy McGruder, two Lean for Life ambassadors who have motivated thousands by going public with their stories.

Thank you, too, to Janet Eastman and Mark Smith, for their editorial insight; to Frank Groff for his savvy, energetic, enterprising work on behalf of Lindora; to Lance Huante and Piazzo Design for consistently spectacular graphic creations; to Mary Grady at KCBS for thinking of Lindora and caring enough about Tommy McGruder to call; to Ashley Gardner at Pandora Productions for always coming through with brilliance and originality on a moment's notice; and to Griffin Publishing Company—especially Bob Howland, Robin Howland, and Richard Burns, Ph.D.—for sharing our enthusiasm and trusting that this wouldn't be "just another diet book."

I'm profoundly grateful to Herman Frankel, M.D., and his partner, Jean Staeheli, of Portland Health Institute. Their collaboration made the whole project more enjoyable and memorable. The energy and ideas that were generated during the days and nights we spent together were gifts I will always treasure. I am fortunate to have them as my "mental trainers" and personal "BioModifiers." They were there for me 100%, and their warmth and wisdom is reflected throughout this book.

Finally, I want to thank Jerry Holderman, my collaborator and partner on this project. Interest and enthusiasm are essential to accomplish anything of value, and Jerry possesses an abundance of both. Together, we've had our share of "special moments." When this project grew larger and took longer than either of us ever anticipated, Jerry was there to prod me along with his wicked wit, always striving to make the finished product the very best it could possibly be. His unique talent in translating mountains of complex material into the inspiring, highly readable book you're holding is truly a testament to Jerry's remarkable "way with words."

Jerry Holderman

This book has been a true collaboration from the very beginning, blending the experience, talent, and perspective of dozens of people who were committed to excellence and determined to achieve nothing less.

Cynthia Stamper Graff's vision and passion are evident on every page of this book. Her commitment to creating a finished product that would truly benefit its readers has been unwavering, and her enthusiasm during the past year has been unabashed. Every project of this magnitude inevitably has at least one "Black Monday," and Cynthia has weathered ours with resilience and grace. I thank her for believing in this project and in me. My respect for her talent and tenacity has only grown during our collaboration.

I also owe a huge personal debt to four other extraordinary people whose vital contributions have helped make this book what it is:

Herman M. Frankel, M.D.— Dozens of times during the writing of this book, Dr. Frankel ended our telephone conversations with, "I'm with you all the way!" He absolutely was, and words can't express how much I value his wisdom and friendship. He is the godfather of this project.

Jean Staeheli— Her keen insights and astonishing creative consistency were as invaluable in generating ideas and clarifying concepts as they were in coaxing this manuscript across the finish line. Jean is the consummate team player, and her ability to nurture and elicit from others their best — whether she's listening or speaking — is a unique gift.

Janet Eastman— Her editorial instincts and wit are every bit as sharp—and appreciated—as the day we met 16 years ago. Janet's willingness to go above and beyond the call of duty on this project only reinforces what I've long known: she's a class act.

Rick Davis— His good humor, generous spirit, thoughtful advice, and consistent support have had a far greater impact on this project—and on me— than he realizes.

I'm deeply grateful, as well, for a small but stalwart circle of close friends whose emotional generosity and extraordinary encouragement makes a difference in my life every day: Ali Fadakar, Kiko Rodriguez, Joyce Pederson, Jack Herzberg, Gary Costa, Ellen McGrath, Ph.D., and Veston Rowe.

Thank you, too, to my family. No matter where they are, they are with me: Ruth Lawrence, Jan Knudten, Daniel Holderman, Dorothy Sebell, Leonard Sebell, Kathy Holderman, Jim Holderman, Rachele Cost, Judy Eratostene, Zelma Dolph, Harold Dolph, Alice Holderman, Gerald Holderman, Nellie Jackson, and Clara Dutch Spalding.

I also thank Dr. Marshall Stamper for generously sharing his wisdom and his knowledge; Nell Stamper, who elevates Southern hospitality to new heights; Diana Rosenfeld, for sharing her heart and soul and for inspiring so many to do so much; and six other special people whose daily commitment to the Lindora program and the people it serves was apparent every time we talked—Peter Vash, M.D., Jan Hunter, R.N., Debbie Riley, L.V.N., Jayme Davidson, R.N., Susan Adams, L.V.N., and Lynne Nieto, N.P.

Frank Groff helped get the ball rolling—thank you, Frank, for the vote of confidence and for making the connection. Thanks, too, to the management at Griffin Publishing Company—Bob Howland, Robin Howland, and Richard Burns, Ph.D.—for seeing the potential of this project and for doing their best to maximize it.

I also value the enormous creative contribution that Lance Huante and the entire crew at Piazzo Design—especially Dan Webster and David Salmassian— have made to the look and feel of the finished product. Their collective sense of taste and style is equalled only by their patience. And special thanks to Ingrid Herman Reese and Michael Hendrickson, whose spirit of collaboration and attention to detail under daunting deadline pressure makes their contribution to this project all the more impressive and appreciated.

Many others have also supported me along the way through their words and actions. My thanks to Edward Abraham, M.D., Frank Alcala, Joksan Alcala at The MacEnthusiasts in Los Angeles, Richard Ammon, Ph.D., Patricia Bell, William J. Bell, Michael Bertsch, Kate Navin Booth, William Brown, Michelle Clark, Rev. Gary Davis, Belinda DeLong, Steven Fisher, Daniel Franco, Agnes Griffith, Moana Grochow, Nigel Hampton, Ph.D., Jack Hanson, Dee Dee Hanson, Megan Hodges, Joyce Hoffspiegel, Ph.D., John Humphrey, Maxine Humphrey, Carolyn Johnson, Jeff Kaufman, Marc LaFont, Melody Lucero, Jay Marzullo, Jamie O'Brien Moore, Olivia Moreno, William Nagel, Mary Beth Nelson, Gary Parsons, Trena Parsons, C.J. Platania, Michael Platania, Jeanne Reiss, Ron Russell, Ph.D., Hooman Shirian at Barbara's Place, Mark Smith, Scott McBride Smith, Gwen Stewart, Duncan Strauss, Cheryl Thompson, Patty Thompson, Jerry Thompson, Joyce Ukropina, Cynthia Vartan, Javier Villalobos, and Harry Wexler, Ph.D.

And, of course, Charlotte, who was there every step of the way.

FOREWORD

Although hundreds of weight-loss programs and diet books have come and gone over the past 35 years, Americans today are fatter than ever. Back in 1961, about 25% of the population was obese. In 1996, that figure had increased to nearly 34%. One of every three men and women in the United States weighs more than 20% above his or her ideal body weight.

This striking increase isn't the result of any alteration in genetic factors. No one's DNA has changed. And while life and the way we live it is unquestionably different from the way it once was, the basic structure of our lives is not. Back then, people had jobs, attended school, played sports, raised kids, and went to the movies. We still do.

What has changed, however, is the way many of us have chosen to react to the rapidly changing, increasingly stressful environment in which we live. While you may not be able to pinpoint exactly why you've gained weight, you can do something to change it. You possess the power to regain your health, dignity, and future, and the support and guidance this book provides can help you do it. You can lose weight. You can learn how to maintain your weight within a safe, healthy range. You can become Lean for Life.

I was first introduced to the Lindora Medical Clinics and the Lean for Life program in 1990, when, as president of the American Society of Bariatric Physicians, I was asked to give a presentation to the company's medical staff. What impressed me most about the people at Lindora was their deep-rooted commitment to the principles of compassionate patient care and the apparent results they were achieving.

When I first reviewed the Lindora program, it struck me as sensible, safe, and effective. It was devoid of hype and supported with solid scientific merit. The program is built upon a medically sound, common-sense foundation. Once you understand and apply its principles, you can be confident in your ability to not only lose your excess fat, but to keep it off.

The weight-loss principles on which the Lean for Life program is based have stood the test of time for more than a quarter-century, helping hundreds of thousands of obese people regain control of their bodies and their lives. The program continues to be just as effective today. Few of the "breakthrough" diets, best-selling diet books, or self-styled diet-and-fitness gurus are around or even remembered after a few years, but Lindora has been and will continue to be.

As Executive Medical Director of Lindora, my responsibility is to bring to the program new scientific advances that will enhance safe and effective weight loss. While the field of obesity treatment continues to be filled with quack remedies and bogus professionals promising miracle cures, the Lean for Life program continues to incorporate only the soundest of scientific principles.

This is a book about change—changing the way you eat, feel, think, look, and live. It's about investing in your own health and happiness. Anyone who uses this book on their weight-loss journey can be assured of having a responsible, reliable guide.

—Peter Vash, M.D., M.P.H.
Former President, American Society of Bariatric Physicians
Assistant Clinical Professor, UCLA School of Medicine
Executive Medical Director, Lindora Medical Clinics

1

LEAN FOR LIFE

You are beginning a personal journey of self-discovery and self-improvement.

It was showtime. As a burst of applause and the show's lively theme music filled the room, television talk show host Maury Povich made his entrance. He stopped center stage, stared into one of the cameras and began sharing a story that instantly riveted the audience.

"When we first met Diana Rosenfeld," Povich began, "she needed an oversized wheelchair and a freight elevator just to make it into our studios."

As a montage of video clips showed astonishing images of Diana struggling to walk, he explained that she had once weighed even more—641 pounds.

"Just getting around had become a major production," Povich continued, "and she tried just about everything to lose weight. Diana was desperate. She had to do something. Finally, she found the Lindora Clinic.... It was working. Diana's last-ditch diet was paying off."

Povich briskly recapped her three previous visits on the show while powerful photographs of a steadily shrinking Diana appeared on the studio monitors.

"I remember Diana well when she was 641 pounds, 409 pounds and 316 pounds. I wonder what she looks like now? I haven't seen her since she came to our studio today on this trip to New York. Now everyone, let's please welcome...the new Diana Rosenfeld."

On cue, Diana emerged. She looked radiant. More to the point, she looked healthy. Povich shrieked with delight when a beaming Diana stopped mid-stage and did a spontaneous twirl to show off her new body. As she confidently strolled past her lifesize "before" picture and toward the host's open arms, the audience sprang to its feet.

More than a few of the onlookers were moved to tears. I was one of them. I couldn't help but remember the day I first met Diana. Was this animated, vibrant woman standing on stage in a Manhattan television studio really the same person who had struggled through our front door at the Lindora Medical Clinics in Costa Mesa, California just three years earlier?

Over the years, from my first job with Lindora as a 19-year-old medical assistant through today in my present position as its president,

A Lean for Life Success Story

DIANA ROSENFELD:

THEN&NOW

"I was never an unattractive woman— just well hidden. I've lost more than 400 pounds on the Lean for Life program. In the process, I've gained a degree of self-esteem and self-respect that is helping me redefine my life."

I've met thousands of overweight people. Diana was, without question, the largest woman I had ever met. None of the clinicians at Lindora had ever worked with anyone her size, but that was no reason for us not to. While a majority of the people who do our medically supervised weight-control program want to lose between 30 and 60 pounds, we had been successful in helping many people lose between 100 and 250 pounds.

At 641 pounds, Diana had two choices: to lose weight or die. Other doctors and programs had declined to work with her, writing her off as a lost cause. But we believed we could help her. We knew that Diana's goal to lose weight was realistic and achievable. We also knew that our program, which has evolved over 25 years and five million patient treatments, is scientifically sound and would be safe and healthy for her. What's more, we knew that if she followed it, it would generate the results she said she wanted. The only unknown was whether Diana possessed the desire, commitment, and level of enthusiasm it takes to achieve any goal.

She certainly did. As her weight melted away, Diana's spirits soared. She soon became a goodwill ambassador for Lindora, sharing her success story on television and radio shows all over the world. Her story appeared in magazines and newspapers nationally and internationally. She was, as they say, "hot copy."

With each new television appearance or newspaper story, interest in Diana and our weight-loss program escalated. Thousands of phone calls, some from as far away as Japan, England, and Egypt, flooded our switchboard. We even received a call from one of the entertainment industry's best known stars, wondering whether we'd consider opening our clinic near Beverly Hills early every morning so she could slip in and out undetected on her way to the studio.

"ANYTHING YOU COULD SEND ME IS A LOT MORE THAN I HAVE RIGHT NOW"

Stacks—sometimes bags—of "fan mail" arrived for Diana nearly every day. Whether the letters were postmarked from Seattle or Shreveport, there was a common thread in every one of their stories: a sense of hope that if Diana could do it, they could, too. What people wanted, pure and simple, was the program Diana used. "Anything you could send me," wrote a woman from Detroit, "is a lot more than I have right now."

While the enormous outpouring of interest was heartening, it was also frustrating. Every letter and call reminded us that behind the statistics—60 million Americans are obese; one of every three adults in

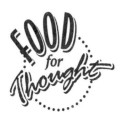

"It's never too late

to be who you

might have been."

— George Eliot

this country weighs more than 20% above his or her ideal body weight—there are real people searching for real solutions. But since our program was offered exclusively in a clinical setting, we couldn't help anyone who wasn't able to visit one of our Southern California clinics.

Or could we? Was it possible to take a complex program that was currently being provided by trained nurses and doctors in our clinics and simplify it without compromising safety, quality, or results? It was essential not only that people do the program safely and comfortably, but that they achieve results comparable to those our patients had come to expect.

"AT HOME...BUT NOT ALONE"

We launched a Lindora "At Home...But Not Alone" program to explore the possibilities. For more than 12 months, we worked with men and women ranging in age from 24 to 68. Some lived thousands of miles away. Each received an instruction manual that was far less comprehensive than this book, along with a package of support products that included audio tapes, a step counter, vitamins, and an assortment of medical-grade protein supplements to be used in addition to a healthy menu of lean meats, vegetables, and fruits. We monitored their progress by telephone.

Within nine months, the verdict was in. The program was a success. People throughout the country were enjoying impressive results. Ron, a computer programmer from Dumfries, Virginia, lost 102 pounds. Candice, a 24-year-old hotel executive living in New York City, dropped 30 pounds. Stan, a Mississippi newspaper editor, lost 49 pounds and recovered from major surgery faster than his doctors expected.

And then there was Tommy McGruder. In May 1995, we received a call from Mary Grady, a television news reporter from KCBS, the CBS affiliate in Los Angeles. She explained that a man weighing more than 800 pounds had been carried out of his house by 11 firefighters and taken to the USC Medical Center. He was in respiratory distress and was literally being crushed to death by his excess weight.

Grady, whose station had done several stories on Diana Rosenfeld, wondered if anything could be done for Tommy. Though he lived just a few miles from our Inglewood clinic, Tommy had been bedridden for two years, unable to walk. He would need to be treated through our "At Home...But Not Alone" program.

On May 8, 1996, Tommy McGruder celebrated one year on the program. So far, he has lost more than 450 pounds. Tommy's experience was yet another validation that we had successfully developed a way to provide the at-home guidance and support so many thousands of people had sought.

As you read this book, you won't be alone, either. While it can't duplicate the support our patients receive from trained professionals in our clinics, this book is your gateway to a number of valuable resources, including Lindora's site on the World Wide Web, our bimonthly newsletter, the audio tapes, video tapes, and print materials we make available to our patients, as well as our telephone resource center, where you can get answers to questions you may have along the way.

THE LEAN FOR LIFE ADVANTAGE

As you'll discover, *Lean for Life* is much more than a book about how to lose weight. It's a book about change: changing the way you eat, the way you look, the way you feel, and the way you think. It's a comprehensive, personalized program in which you'll discover how your self-image and your relationship with food have led to the weight problem you've decided to address. You will *gain* awareness as you *lose* weight. You'll learn how to become Lean for Life. And most important, you'll learn how to *stay* that way.

While writing this book, we asked Lindora patients for suggestions. One woman, a patient in our Laguna Hills clinic, was adamant: "Spare me a lot of theory. Just show me how to lose the weight and show me how to keep it off!"

That's exactly what this book does. *Lean for Life* guides you through a straightforward, results-oriented program designed to help you lose weight rapidly, safely, and comfortably. One month from today, you can easily weigh 15 pounds less than you do right now—and you can repeat the weight-loss phase of the program until you lose all the weight you want!

THE THREE-PHASE APPROACH TO BECOMING—AND STAYING—LEAN FOR LIFE

The Lean for Life program is divided into three phases: Weight Loss, Metabolic Adjustment, and Lifetime Maintenance. You'll do all three phases while eating healthy, nutritious food from the grocery store.

"Phase 1: Weight Loss" lasts 28 days or less, depending on your weight-loss goal. During Phase 1, you'll be limiting your calories and your intake of carbohydrates—your body's primary energy source—so that your body will rely on its alternate energy system, body fat, for energy.

THE LEAN FOR LIFE PROGRAM: AN OVERVIEW

THE "PREP"— 1-3 DAYS

A period of one to three days during which you prepare your body and your mind for "Phase 1: Weight Loss."

"PHASE 1: WEIGHT LOSS"— 28 DAYS

After completing a three-day preparation or "prep diet," you will begin "Phase 1: Weight Loss," which lasts 28 days (or less, depending on your weight-loss goal). Each 28-day weight-loss period is called a "series."

Week 1	Days 1-3	Protein Days
	Days 4-7	Weight-Loss Menu Days
Week 2	Day 8	Protein Day
	Days 9-14	Weight-Loss Menu Days
Week 3	Day 15	Protein Day
	Days 16-21	Weight-Loss Menu Days
Week 4	Day 22	Protein Day
	Days 23-28	Weight-Loss Menu Days

After completing a maximum of 28 days on "Phase 1: Weight Loss," you'll move directly into "Phase 2" Metabolic Adjustment"—even if you want to lose more weight.

"PHASE 2: METABOLIC ADJUSTMENT"—14 DAYS

Day 1	Protein Day
Days 2-3	Metabolic Adjustment, Level 1
Days 4-7	Metabolic Adjustment, Level 2
Day 8	Protein Day
Days 9-14	Metabolic Adjustment, Level 3

Once you've successfully completed "Phase 2: Metabolic Adjustment," you'll have a decision to make. If you want to lose more weight, you can begin another weight-loss series of up to 28 days, followed by another Metabolic Adjustment phase. If you've achieved your weight-loss goal, you'll proceed directly from "Phase 2: Metabolic Adjustment" to "Phase 3: Lifetime Maintenance."

"PHASE 3: LIFETIME MAINTENANCE"

In the three to six months following completion of "Phase 2: Metabolic Adjustment," you'll gradually add a variety of foods to your diet. You'll learn how to achieve "equilibrium" and stabilize at your new lean weight so that you'll be able to eat normally without gaining weight.

As anyone who has ever dieted knows, *losing* weight is only the first step. The challenge is *keeping* it off, which is exactly what the second phase of the program is designed to help you achieve.

After *each* weight-loss series you choose to do, you will move on to "Phase 2: Metabolic Adjustment." During this 14-day period, you'll be increasing your body's metabolism—the rate at which you burn calories—by gradually adding selected foods to your eating plan. Phase 2 is carefully structured to help you retain the results you've achieved during the weight-loss phase. When it's done properly, you will adjust your metabolism *without* experiencing a weight gain.

Once you've lost all the weight you want to lose and have successfully completed "Phase 2: Metabolic Adjustment," you'll graduate to "Phase 3: Lifetime Maintenance." This phase is as vital to your success as the two earlier phases of the program. During Phase 3, the goal is specific: to adjust your setpoint to your new leaner weight so that you can begin to eat normally without gaining weight.

The eating plan and success strategies featured in this book have been refined over time. Since 1971, Lindora nurses and doctors have worked exclusively with overweight people, logging more than five million patient treatments. This book represents what we've learned along the way and presents it in a daily format that's easy to follow and fun to do. As you move through the program day by day, you'll experience for yourself how the knowledge, awareness, and skills you gain will support you in becoming—and staying—Lean for Life!

A PERSONAL JOURNEY

The beauty of the program is that for every success story as compelling as Diana Rosenfeld's or Tommy McGruder's, there are thousands of people just like you who have succeeded in losing 10, 25, or 50 pounds.

Throughout every page of this book, my goal is to be your guide, to lead you on a journey that will be both enlightening and effective. During this process, I'll share with you dozens of stories of people who were once where you are now, wondering how to begin the program and what to expect.

At Lindora, we've learned much of what we know from the experience and stories of real people. But there's one person's story that's especially close to my heart. If it weren't for her, it's unlikely this program would exist.

A few weeks after I first started working on this book, I was sitting at my dining room table, surrounded by reference material. But rather than sifting through the research, I found myself staring out the window and thinking about my Grandma Angie, the woman whose

THE BENEFITS OF THE LEAN FOR LIFE PROGRAM

If you've ever tried traditional dieting—and who hasn't?—you know what an uphill struggle it can be. You think about food and are nagged by cravings. You often feel sluggish or irritable. And if and when you *do* lose weight, it's typically a slow, tedious process.

On the Lean for Life program, you'll lose weight rapidly, burning excess body fat as fuel at the fastest rate possible while maintaining your lean muscle mass. What's more, you'll have fewer cravings and feel less hungry, less often. You'll experience increased energy and feel terrific!

LEAN FOR LIFE	TRADITIONAL DIETING
Rapid weight loss	Slow weight loss
Reduced hunger	Increased hunger
Fewer cravings	More cravings
Increased energy	Decreased energy
Elevated mood	Often irritable
Maintain lean muscle mass	Lose muscle as well as fat

battle with obesity inspired my father, Dr. Marshall B. Stamper, to begin what was to become Lindora Medical Clinics.

My grandmother was a bosomy, robust woman with a rich Southern drawl, a big laugh, and an even bigger heart. For as long as I could remember, she had always been a very large woman. Once, when I couldn't have been more than five or six years old, I was sitting on the bed as she undressed. I had never seen her without a dress on and I remember being mesmerized by her mammoth thighs.

I was too young at the time to understand the health risks associated with carrying so many extra pounds, just as I was too young to know where the pounds came from in the first place.

Grandma Angie was a fabulous cook and I loved watching her prepare one of her specialties—large, soft, white pieces of fat fried in a heavy, blackened iron skillet. I can still taste the crisp, bacony pieces of fat and the squares of fried bread that she prepared in the leftover liquid fat.

Unfortunately, not all my memories of my grandmother are as pleasant. One Christmas Eve, several years later, the holiday spirit was shattered when she nearly died of congestive heart failure. I remember feeling totally helpless as the ambulance pulled away, its shrill siren fading into the night. Not too long after that, my grandmother died from complications of obesity.

I know all too well the toll that excess weight can take. I'm the granddaughter of a wonderful woman who died too soon because she ate too much. I'm the daughter of a man whose passion for helping overweight people has had a major impact in shaping the way I think about diet, health, and fitness. I'm the mother of a four-year-old daughter, determined to raise her with a healthy body—and a healthy body image—in a culture that reveres frightfully thin models as the feminine ideal. I'm also someone who lost weight on the program 25 years ago and who continues to practice its principles to maintain my weight today. I'm passionate about this program and am proud and delighted to be able to share it with you.

CREATING YOUR OWN SUCCESS STORY

This book is a collaborative effort in the truest sense of the word. It's not only a collaboration among the thousands of Lindora patients and "Team Lindora" employees whose wisdom and personal experience it reflects, but ultimately it's a collaboration between us. You. And me. That's because *Lean for Life* is not simply a book you *read*. It's a book you *do*. And until *you* make it come to life by doing the program it provides, it's merely paragraphs on a page.

The most important story has yet to be written. It's yours. Unlike a novel, in which the author's imagination determines the fate of the main character, how this book ends is ultimately up to you. It's *your* success story—one *you* are about to create.

The first step is turning the page.

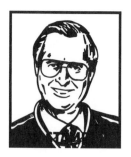

"I call them the 'Six Essentials' because I'm convinced that once you understand these concepts and master them, you'll never again need to diet. You will truly be Lean for Life."

THE SIX ESSENTIALS

What distinguishes those who succeed from those who don't? Over the years, Dr. Marshall Stamper, founder of the Lindora Medical Clinics, has noted that Lindora patients who succeed in losing weight—and maintaining their weight loss—engage in a number of strategies that clearly contribute to their success on the program. Can you do it? It's time to **DECIDE**:

Discover: Before you can become Lean for Life, it's essential to learn how. The learning process is all about discovering bits and pieces of information that result in "Aha! moments": those exciting times when you "get it," when you say to yourself, "*Now* I understand how that applies to me," "I now see how I can do it *differently*," or "*That's* why that's important!"

Enthuse: Generating feelings of enthusiasm, excitement, and energy is essential for achieving nearly anything in life, especially losing weight. Studies of Olympic athletes, world-class musicians, and long-term weight-loss maintainers show that an ability to consistently maintain a high level of interest is one of the greatest factors that distinguishes the best from the rest.

Control Cravings: To control your weight it's essential to learn to control cravings. On the program, you'll discover the various causes of cravings and learn how to overcome them.

Integrate: To become lean and stay lean, the changes you've made to get the results you want must become a permanent part of your life. Without integrating those changes, you're likely to regain the weight you've lost.

Disarm Barriers: Achieving your weight-loss goal requires change, and change isn't easy. In fact, it can be challenging and sometimes even painful. To be successful, you must recognize your "internal barriers" and learn to disarm them.

Exercise: Food is fuel. To become and stay Lean for Life, it's essential that you exercise regularly so that you *burn* fuel rather than store it.

2

THE STARTING LINE

*You will have everything you need
to reach your goal.*

While every person who chooses to do this program shares a common goal—to become Lean for Life—the path you travel is yours alone. In the coming weeks, you'll have many opportunities to look at the big picture as well as the details of your life. You'll clarify what works for you and what you'd like to change.

Together, we'll be doing important work. By the time you finish this book, you will have lost a significant amount of weight. You'll understand why conventional diets don't work and how you've contributed to your own frustration in your previous efforts to lose weight. You'll also become as knowledgeable as the best-informed scientists and clinicians about the ways in which your body gains and loses fat, and how you can tip the scale in your favor. You'll discover what works and, just as important, what doesn't.

So today's the day! You're about to set out on an empowering journey of weight loss, self-improvement, and self-discovery that will result in your looking better, feeling healthier, and being more fully equipped than ever to meet whatever challenges life offers you.

For some, today represents an exciting new beginning, a fresh start. They will experience a renewed sense of focus and a stronger

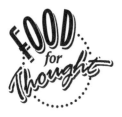

commitment to themselves. They will see it as a great adventure and will be eager to seize the day.

For others, the day brings with it an element of apprehension. Having lost weight in the past, only to regain it, they're more likely to be cautiously optimistic. They believe in the program, sometimes more than they believe in themselves, and are willing to "try it," but they won't be entirely convinced it will "work" for them until they do it.

How are *you* feeling right now? Are you enthusiastic? Ambivalent? Afraid? Whatever emotions you're experiencing, *what ultimately matters isn't what you're feeling but what you're doing.* You've chosen to make something positive happen for yourself, and you've already taken some major steps.

Where will this new path take you? What will happen along the way? Envision yourself on a spectacular hilltop, sitting comfortably beneath a tree. The air is clean and the view is majestic. The warmth of the afternoon sun is tempered by a gentle breeze. An occasional bird call is the only sound you notice. A rolling field of fragrant, colorful flowers is framed by a lush forest. Far in the distance, snow-capped mountains pierce the clear blue sky.

Winding down the hill is a trail your eyes can follow for several hundred yards. The trail begins to twist and turn, eventually fading into the forest. Although you can't see the end, you know that when you begin traveling down that trail, you will always be able to see far enough ahead to continue moving safely. You're comfortable with the thought that you have the rest of your life to follow the trail to its end. You know that the adventures you encounter along the way are the story of your life.

It doesn't matter whether you've been down other trails before. Your journey to becoming Lean for Life will be different, because you will decide how far you want to go and how quickly you want to get there. You will learn how to get back on the path if you happen to lose your way.

Along the way, remember three things:

1. You're making this journey *for* yourself, but not *by* yourself. This book will be your companion and supporter along the way, as will the men and women who will share their stories with you. You'll also have access to a support system that can include our clinical staff, our World World Web site on the Internet, and telephone support.

2. You will accomplish your goal of better health and a better body, but not by doing the same things you've done in the past. You will learn to travel lighter, leaving behind the baggage of past dieting experiences and picking up new tools, strategies, and techniques.

3. You have the time you need to accomplish all you want. You're beginning a lifelong journey where quick fixes don't exist. Establishing new habits takes time. You know that you can maintain your pace as you work for lasting change.

This book is designed to guide you, day-by-day, through the program, introducing new ideas and information along the way. What you learn tomorrow will build upon what you learn today. We know from clinical experience that most people find it much easier to learn and apply new information when they are exposed to it gradually. We call this learning process the "drip method." So rather than being flooded with chapters of concepts and theory before you have an understanding of how to apply any of it, you'll see step-by-step exactly where you're going and how the knowledge you gain each day will help get you there.

If you fall behind on your reading on any given day, don't panic or get discouraged. Simply make a note to read those pages the following day. It's also a good idea to review the material from earlier days as you continue through the program. Patients often comment that they're amazed at how much good information they missed the first time through.

You're ready, so let's get started. The view from here is beautiful. Even more beautiful vistas await you on the path.

FACING THE FEAR

Fear of failure. It's the single most common reason for not starting a weight-loss program. If you've ever dieted and not lost weight—or regained whatever weight you did lose—some degree of apprehension is natural.

The question is how to deal with that fear. Will you manage it or will it manage you? It's easy to let fear surface in the form of excuses: "I'm too stressed and busy to start anything new right now," "I always gain it back anyway, so what's the point?", "I don't really feel that bad." But will statements like these help you achieve your weight-loss goal?

The Lean for Life program offers a rare opportunity for you to practice life-management skills while losing weight. Take the time to read several of the "Lean for Life Success Stories" featured throughout the book. You can be sure every one of these people experienced episodes of fear and self-doubt along the way. And yet they did it. They were determined to overcome the fear of failure in order to earn the pride of accomplishment. They succeeded. You can, too.

PREP DAY 1

PREPARING FOR THE PROGRAM

You'll learn how to effectively prepare
for the weight-loss phase of the program.

Before you begin the weight-loss phase of the Lean for Life program, it's important that you prepare or "prep" for the next three days. The purpose of the Prep is to get your mind and body ready to accomplish your goal. Our clinic nurses tell us that patients who begin their program with a good Prep tend to feel better and achieve greater results during the weight-loss phase of the program.

The Prep serves several purposes. It provides a comfortable transition into "dieting," especially for those whose eating habits have been undisciplined and unstructured. It also offers an opportunity for you to satisfy any lingering cravings before you begin the program.

If you've been dieting and restricting your calories for two weeks or more, the Prep can help replenish your body's reserves of essential fatty acids and amino acids. What's more, the Prep may be beneficial in helping to allow for gallbladder contraction. Research studies suggest there may be a small, temporary increased risk for the development of gallstones in overweight or obese patients during weight loss. This appears to be related to the absence, over a period of time, of a small but necessary amount of fat in the diet that allows for gallbladder contraction. A good Prep helps provide that fat. Throughout the weight-loss phase, you will also be eating foods that contain adequate but reduced amounts of fat, which help to reduce the risk of gallbladder disease.

If you have, or have had, any history that suggests gallbladder disease (attacks of sharp pain in your right upper abdomen, usually accompanied by nausea, gas and/or bloating after eating), be sure to discuss your symptoms with your doctor. It's important to be aware of the risks associated with weight loss and to carefully monitor any physical symptoms.

HOW TO PREP

1. During the three-day Prep, be sure to eat at least three complete meals a day. Your meals should include a protein food, a salad with dressing, a potato, vegetables, fresh fruit, and milk or the calorie-free beverage of your choice. Make sure your between-meal snacks are protein-based — foods such as cheese, nuts, seeds, celery with peanut butter, yogurt. Review the Sample "Prep Day" Menu on the following page for examples of food choices.

   If there are certain foods you sometimes crave but try to avoid, such as pizza or cheeseburgers, for example, you may have them now. The Prep is not an excuse to "pig out," yet it is an opportunity to satisfy any nagging cravings before beginning the weight-loss phase of the program. Do your best to avoid or limit candy, cakes, cookies, pies, and alcohol, as they can trigger cravings and stimulate your appetite. And use common sense. People who make the mistake of treating the three Prep Days as a "last hurrah" can end up unnecessarily gaining as much as 10 pounds. Why set the starting line back when you don't need to?

2. Begin taking two vitamin/mineral supplements (Lean for Life or equivalent), three times a day, after each meal. (See page 35.)

3. Begin drinking 80 ounces of water or other calorie-free beverages a day. (Three 32-ounce squeezable sports bottles make it easy to remember how much water you're drinking.)

4. Continue with any exercise program you currently follow.

GETTING IT TOGETHER: YOUR RECIPE FOR SUCCESS

To prepare for the weight-loss phase of the program, you'll need to gather these "ingredients" over the next few days. These items can be purchased at most drug or discount stores; many may be ordered through the Resources section.

- ❑ Ketone-measuring sticks
- ❑ Food scale
- ❑ Measuring cups and spoons
- ❑ Water bottle (30 oz. or larger)
- ❑ Weight scale
- ❑ Tape measure
- ❑ Pedometer (step counter)
- ❑ Cassette player
- ❑ Blank cassette tape
- ❑ Your food shopping list

SAMPLE "PREP DAY" DIET

BREAKFAST
2 eggs or omelette
Bacon, ham, or sausage (if desired)
1 slice whole wheat toast with butter
6-8 ounces unsweetened orange juice

LUNCH
Tuna salad sandwich, chicken salad sandwich,
    or pizza
Green salad with dressing
Fresh fruit
Coffee or any calorie-free beverage

DINNER
6 ounces steak or fish
Baked potato with butter and sour cream
Green salad with dressing
Fresh fruit or other dessert
Coffee or any calorie-free beverage

SNACKS
Cheese, nuts, seeds, celery with peanut butter,
    yogurt

Your Turn

You've made the decision. You're determined to make it happen—no matter what—and you're ready to create a Plan of Action. So now what? Take a few minutes to identify and prioritize your reasons for becoming Lean for Life.

The first challenge is to stay focused. This isn't always easy, because there may be a part of you that raises every possible excuse to keep you from facing the challenge of making changes.

It's important for you to identify your "urgency factor." What was the "final straw" that motivated you to lose weight this time? Often, it's a specific incident, comment, or personal observation that inspires us to make changes.

For Kathy, it was being asked when her baby was due—even though she wasn't pregnant. For Ben, it was having his daughter wonder why his face turned red and he breathed so hard every time he climbed the stairs. For Joan, it was the realization she had worn the same two outfits to work every day for nearly three weeks because all her other clothes no longer fit. What's *your* reason for choosing to make a change in your weight at this time?

Take a moment to complete the following statement:

I decided it was time to do something about my weight when

_____

_____

Now sit down with a stack of 3 x 5 note cards or small sheets of paper. On each card, jot down one benefit you'll enjoy after achieving your weight-loss goal. How will losing weight enhance your self image? How will others see you? Will it benefit you at work? Make it less fatiguing to play with your kids? Here are a few ideas to help get you started:

"I'll be proud of how I look."
"I will feel more in control."
"I could make love with the lights on."
"I would be able to tuck my shirt in."
"I'll be more active with my kids."
"I can play tennis again."
"I'll look terrific at the reunion."

After you've written down all the reasons you can think of, prioritize them. Move the cards around until you've clarified your top five reasons for losing weight, then list them on the following page.

MY PERSONAL MOTIVATORS: HOW I'LL BENEFIT BY BECOMING LEAN FOR LIFE

1. _____

_____

2. _____

_____

3. _____

_____

4. _____

_____

5. _____

_____

Copy the above list on three note cards or pieces of paper. Keep one copy in your purse or wallet. Put the second where you're sure to see it every morning—in your medicine chest, on your bathroom mirror, or in your underwear drawer. Keep the third in a desk drawer at the office, on your car dashboard, or in your gym bag. These reminders will help you stay focused on why you're investing the time and energy to lose weight.

Review your Motivator cards daily. Before long, you'll memorize them and can use them to help yourself maneuver around the inevitable temptations that are sure to come up. When you feel like swinging by the bakery instead of the gym, for example, take a look at your card. Once you do, you'll be much more inclined to think twice and to say "Not so fast!" When you find yourself wondering, "What's wrong with a donut every now and then?" your card has the answer.

ANY QUESTIONS?

Q: *Tell me more about the three Prep Days. I always thought an ideal diet was low in fat.*

A: These three days of relatively higher-fat intake help to insure normal emptying of your gallbladder. This helps protect you from problems that can develop during periods of reduced calorie intake. IMPORTANT: Being overweight increases your risk of gallbladder disease. At the same time, dieting may exacerbate an existing gallbladder condition. If you experience abdominal pain, immediately contact your physician.

Q: *What effect will the three Prep Days have on my cholesterol?*

A: If you normally avoid the kinds of higher-fat foods recommended for prepping, you may experience a minor, temporary increase in your blood cholesterol level. Over the course of the program, however, many people experience a healthy decrease of cholesterol as well as improved HDL (the "good cholesterol").

Chronic high cholesterol can be a health risk. If you have a history of gallbladder or heart disease, consult your doctor before beginning the program to determine whether you're physically able to do the program and if the three Prep Days are necessary. It may be better for you to proceed directly to "Phase 1: Weight Loss."

I NEED HELP   By Vic Lee

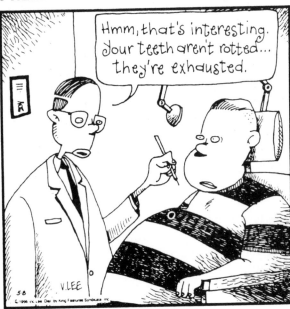

Reprinted with special permission of King Features Syndicate.

PREP DAY 2

MOTIVATING MEASUREMENTS

*You'll discover the importance of setting
goals and measuring your progress.*

The first day of your weight-loss phase of the program is just
around the corner. But before you start, you need to ask
an important question: *"How much weight do I want to lose?"*

This question is one many overweight people would rather avoid.
The more weight people need to lose, the more resistant they will
generally be to declaring a specific long-term weight-loss goal. Instead of
saying, "I will become Lean for Life by losing X pounds," they often
hedge their bets by saying they want to lose "some weight" or that
they want to continue on the program until they "feel healthier" or
"look better."

The problem with such vague goals is that it's virtually impossible
to determine when you've succeeded. Is "some" weight 15 pounds or
50? Is "feeling healthier" being able to tie your shoes without being
short of breath or is it taking a three-hour bike ride on a hot summer day
and living to talk about it? Does "looking better" mean no longer feeling
self-conscious in a pair of shorts or being able to wear your favorite jeans
from college?

Be honest. How much would you like to weigh when you complete "Phase 1: Weight Loss"? If you could blink your eyes and magically transform yourself into a leaner, healthier you, how much would the "new you" weigh? The more clearly you state your goal, the more likely you'll be to achieve it. After all, if you don't know where you want to go, how will you know when you've arrived?

There are a number of ways to determine your "ideal" or "lean" weight. Hydrostatic (underwater) weighing is a highly accurate method for determining your body's composition of lean vs. fat, but it can be expensive and isn't widely available. In our clinics, we use an electrical impedance method that provides computerized calculations of lean weight, standard weight range measurements, and percentage of body fat. People who don't have access to these methods can go to a local gym to have a skinfold thickness test done with simple calipers.

Here are several common-sense measuring techniques you can use at home:

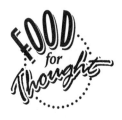

"Never let yesterday use up too much of today."

— Will Rogers

- ❑ *Weigh yourself.* Do you have any idea how much you weighed when you last felt good about your body? If so, a simple bathroom scale can help you estimate an appropriate body weight and monitor your progress.

- ❑ *The proverbial "Rule of Thumb."* Here's another way to establish an "ideal weight." Women: Start with 100 pounds and add five pounds for every inch above five feet. Men: Start at 106 pounds and add six pounds for every inch above five feet.

- ❑ *The pinch test.* Stand up straight. Using your right thumb and index finger, gently squeeze a fold of skin and underlying tissue four inches to the right of your navel. If you can pinch more than a one inch, guess what? You've got fat to spare.

- ❑ *Measure up.* Measure your chest, waist, lower abdomen, hips, and upper thigh. Jot down the numbers below. This is a useful way to monitor fat loss. You'll be doing it again later in the program.

Chest _____

Waist _____

Abdomen _____

Hips _____

Thigh _____

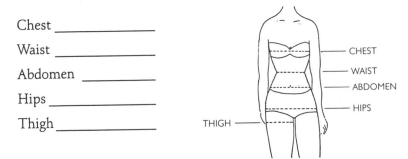

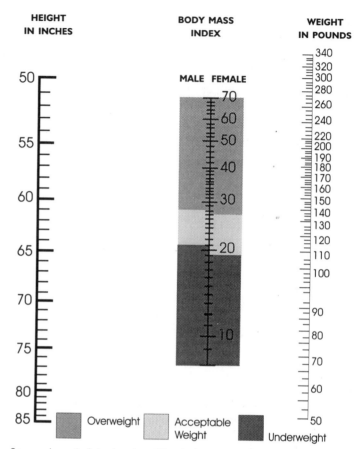

HEIGHT IN INCHES	BODY MASS INDEX	WEIGHT IN POUNDS

Source: *Journal of the American Dietetic Association*, September 1985.

❑ *Calculate your "Body Mass Index."* This is a common measurement used by clinicians to determine health risk factors. This figure, often referred to as your Body Mass Index (BMI), measures your "bigness" or "ponderosity" based on weight and height. The accompanying illustration makes it possible for you to accurately estimate your BMI by drawing a line from your height (on the left side of the illustration) to your weight (on the right). Your BMI is the number at which that line crosses the center. The "acceptable" BMI range for women is between 19 and 25; for men it's between 21 and 26.

❑ *Consult your clothing.* For some people, the snug fit of a favorite pair of pants or skirt is a sure sign it's time to drop a few pounds. If you have clothes that are a little tight around your chest, waist, hips, or thighs, pin a note with today's date on the garment and hang it back in your closet. Jot a reminder on your calendar to try it on again in two weeks and note your progress at that time.

❑ *Take a good look in the mirror.* You may find this one difficult, but it's important to do because it can be a real "reality check." Stand nude in front of a full-length mirror and study the image you see. Is this a body you would choose? Survey various areas. What improvements would you recognize as evidence of weight loss and improved fitness? This is a method you can repeat regularly, setting new goals as you progress.

Remember: Healthy improvement is what's important. It isn't necessary, and in fact may be psychologically unhealthy, to strive for physical "perfection."

❑ *Ask a trusted friend or loved one to help you with an assessment.* It's easy to see what we want to see and to avoid the truth. Ask a trusted friend or loved one to give you a candid assessment of your physical being. Do this only if you think the person can be objective and supportive while sharing these observations.

Be sure to try at least two of these measuring techniques. Then, it's "Your Turn."

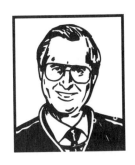

DR. STAMPER

"It's entirely within your power to rethink, reprogram, and redefine the role food plays in your life. The Lean for Life program will show you how. "

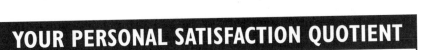

YOUR PERSONAL SATISFACTION QUOTIENT

How you feel about your life—your work, your family, your relationships, your finances, your health, your body— impacts everything you think, say, and do. Are you physically energetic? Are you happy more often than sad? Do you get along with others? Do you like yourself? Circle the number that reflects how you feel about your life *at this moment*:

| 1 | 2 | 3 | 4 | 5 | 6 | 7 | 8 | 9 | 10 |

I've never been more unhappy.   *I'm generally satisfied with my life.*   *My life is terrific!*

We will revisit this question later in the program.

Your Turn

Establish your weight-loss goal.
It's time! Based on what you've just read,
take a few minutes to establish your long-term
weight-loss goal—not how much you want to weigh a
week or a month from now, but what you'd *ideally* like to
weigh. What would that number be if achieving it didn't require
any effort, if you could simply wish it true? Your goal weight is
probably right in that neighborhood. And on this program, you *can*
achieve it— not by "wishing" it true, but by learning and applying the
skills and strategies necessary for becoming and remaining Lean for Life.

My current BMI is _____.

My "Rule of Thumb" ideal weight is _____.

Today I weigh _____ pounds.

My goal weight is _____ pounds

To achieve this goal, I will lose _____ pounds.

I NEED HELP   By Vic Lee

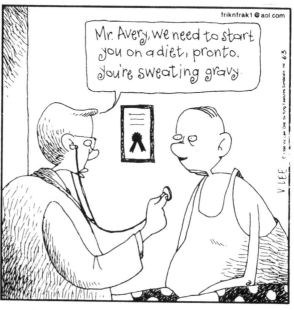

Reprinted with special permission of King Features Syndicate.

Another Lean for Life Success Story

"When I started the program, I said I wanted to lose 50 pounds. I was afraid to tell the truth—that I really wanted to lose 100—because it sounded overwhelming. Then I remembered one of my grandmother's favorite expressions. She used to say that the difference between involvement and commitment was never more obvious than with a bacon-and-egg breakfast. 'The chicken,' she would say, 'was involved, but the pig was committed!' It dawned on me that until I declared my true goal, I was merely involved. Once I did, I became committed, and it's made all the difference in the world. I've lost 87 pounds and I'm still going strong!"

— Rob

PREP DAY 3

THE MIND-BODY CONNECTION

You'll discover how what happens in your mind affects what happens in your body—and vice versa.

Words can make you blush. Jokes can make you laugh. Movies can make you cry. Conversations can make you sweat. A card or call from that special someone can get your heart racing.

The connection between your mind and body is undeniable. The thoughts you think, the emotions you feel, the images you see, and the things you do all affect your behavior and your body chemistry. Likewise, your body chemistry and your behavior affect how you think, how you feel, your impressions of what you see, and what you do.

Only recently have scientists and researchers begun to understand how profound the mind-body connection is, and how you can intentionally use it to achieve specific goals such as weight loss.

Every page of this book reflects the power and potential of the mind-body connection. Our goal is to give you the tools that will make this connection work positively for you.

If you're feeling sorry for yourself, we'll encourage you to do things that will give you pleasure. If just thinking about exercise makes you tired, we'll help you learn to think about it differently. If you're feeling edgy, we'll offer ways to relax. If you're frustrated, we'll share success stories of others who've experienced the same feelings and have overcome them. If you're overwhelmed, we'll suggest ways to refocus your thoughts and energy.

Together we'll explore the importance of treating yourself well, clarifying goals, and cultivating an "achievement attitude." You'll become an effective problem-solver, learn how to mentally rehearse being successful, and understand what you can do to change your body chemistry.

Our patients are often surprised to discover that many successful weight-loss strategies can be learned. You can learn to control cravings, eat lean, and enjoy exercise. You can also learn to feel deserving of—and comfortable with—a more attractive, healthier body.

VISUALIZING YOUR SUCCESS

No matter how enthusiastic you are when you start the program, it's easy to lose momentum once the initial excitement fades. That's why it's vital to have a visual reminder of your goals.

Here are two ideas to help you succeed. Choose whichever appeals to you most or come up with your own motivational idea. Whatever you do, make sure it's a graphic reminder of why you're on the program.

1. *Find an "After" photograph of yourself.* You may have to dig through boxes or photo albums, but find a picture of yourself when you were leaner and healthier. Choose one that captures the physical image you want to project again.

   If you don't have photographs available, thumb through magazines and cut out images of people who look the way you would like to look. Be sure to focus on overall body image rather than the face or hairstyle. And whatever you do, be practical. Don't set yourself up with unrealistic expectations. Nothing can be more demoralizing than comparing yourself to an airbrushed, perfectly lighted image of an actor or model.

   Some people find it valuable to do this exercise with someone they trust to give them honest feedback as to what body type is realistic and appropriate.

2. *Create an "After" picture of yourself.* One woman who succeeded on the program came up with a clever way to visualize her leaner body. Alice asked her daughter to take several photographs of her wearing a one-piece swimsuit. She selected one of the pictures as her "Before" photo and used a second photo from the same session to create her "After" shot.

Alice took a fine-line pen and outlined her leaner, healthier body shape on the photo. Using a pair of manicure scissors, she trimmed away the weight she was determined to lose. With a few snips, she had created an image that motivated her to pursue her goal.

It's your future. Picture it!

HOW STRONG IS THE MIND–BODY CONNECTION?

❑ Susan Everson, an epidemiologist at the Western Consortium for Public Health in Berkeley, California, and her colleagues have shown that men who are depressed die from heart disease, cancer, and other causes at higher than average rates.

❑ Neurologists at the National Institute of Mental Health have found that practicing a physical skill for just a few minutes a day alters the brain, dramatically increasing one's ability to perform the task. The more one practices a task, the more developed the relevant area of the brain becomes.

❑ Richard Restak, M.D., author of *Brainscapes*, reports numerous instances of behavior affecting brain structure. Blind people who study Braille, for example, develop a larger area of the brain assigned to the use of the left index finger, the finger that "reads" Braille text.

3

"PHASE 1: WEIGHT LOSS" OVERVIEW OF THE FIRST WEEK

After you finish this brief introduction, which also includes the menu plan, you'll immediately begin taking action to become Lean for Life by moving directly into Day 1 of "Phase 1: Weight Loss."

Phase 1 lasts 28 days and begins with three days that are referred to as "Protein Days." The menus for the special "Protein Days" feature high-protein, low-calorie, low-carbohydrate food choices geared to jump-starting your body into burning fat for fuel.

Whenever you sufficiently restrict your intake of carbohydrates—your body's primary energy source—for a long enough period of time, you'll reach a point where your body starts using its own alternate energy system, fat stores, for energy. This means your body mobilizes your stored fat and burns it for fuel. This process results in the production of ketone bodies, which appear in your urine. In other words, you recycle your stored body fat. Body fat, which was once food, becomes fuel again!

Throughout Phase 1, you'll know whether you're burning fat, and are therefore "in ketosis," because you'll be monitoring your urine with a ketone-measuring strip or "ketostick" every morning. Jan Hunter,

Lindora's Director of Nursing, refers to these ketone sticks as the "FBI"—Fat Burning Indicators.

As significant amounts of fat stores are burned, ketone bodies are produced, causing the ketostick to change color. You want to achieve "good color"—a range from lavender to deep purple. If it *doesn't* change color, you'll know you've consumed too many carbohydrates during a recent meal or snack and you will know how to make immediate adjustments in your eating plan.

Lindora patients tell us they like this aspect of the program because it provides objective confirmation that the program is working. If you already have your ketosticks, you might want to test your urine now. Since you haven't started the weight-loss menu, it's unlikely that you'll "show color" yet. But at least you'll have a point of reference. You'll know what a negative result looks like. You'll also reinforce the knowledge that when you're not following the plan, your ketostick will be negative. Remember this for the future.

Our patients lose between two and five pounds per week during Weight Loss. The amount you lose can be influenced by individual variables such as age, gender, starting weight, level of activity, and how carefully you follow the program. *If you don't lose all the weight you want to lose during your first cycle through Phase 1, you can repeat the process until you achieve your Lean for Life goal.* Repeating the process means up to four more weeks of "Phase 1: Weight Loss," followed by another two weeks of "Phase 2: Metabolic Adjustment." You can repeat this six-week process until you reach your lean weight, at which point you will begin "Phase 3: Lifetime Maintenance."

CATHY   **By Cathy Guisewite**

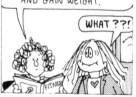

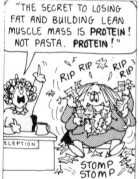

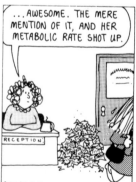

YOUR LEAN FOR LIFE "PHASE I: WEIGHT LOSS" MENU PLAN

BEGIN THIS AFTER YOUR PROTEIN DAYS (usually Day 4)

During "Phase I: Weight Loss," you'll be paying attention to the number of grams of carbohydrate in the food you choose, as well as how much and how often you're eating. Following is your Lean for Life "Phase I: Weight Loss" Menu Plan:

BREAKFAST
1 meat/protein
1 fruit *or* 1 grain
Choice of any calorie-free beverage

MORNING SNACK
Choice of one serving from the Protein list.

LUNCH
1 meat/protein
1 vegetable
1 fruit
2 cups, torn lettuce
Salad dressing (choice of any nonfat
   product, up to 15 calories and
   3 grams carbohydrate)
Choice of any calorie-free beverage

AFTERNOON SNACK
Choice of one serving from the Protein list.

DINNER
1 meat/protein
1 vegetable
1 fruit
2 cups, torn lettuce
Salad dressing (choice of any nonfat
   product, up to 15 calories and
   3 grams carbohydrate)
Choice of any calorie-free beverage

EVENING SNACK
Choice of one serving from the Protein list.

MISCELLANEOUS
Your choice of one serving, twice per day, with the meals of your choice:

Gelatin (diet)	1/2 cup
Green onion (tops)	1 tsp.
Horseradish	1 tsp.
Jalapeño Pepper	2 small
Margarine (nonfat)	1 Tbs. (5 cal. maximum)
Mustard	1 tsp.
Pimento	1 tsp.
Radishes	2 medium
Vinegar (unseasoned)	2 Tbs.

BEVERAGES
Water
Coffee*
Decaffeinated coffee
Tea (hot or iced)*
Herbal tea
Diet soda*
Diet seltzer
Diet mineral water
Any other calorie-free drink

*This beverage may contain caffeine, which tends to stimulate appetite and may make you feel jumpy or "wired." If you choose drinks containing caffeine, you may want to limit them. Rely on decaffeinated beverages between meals. If you reduce or eliminate caffeine, do it *gradually*. Coffee lovers and anyone used to drinking tea and soda can experience withdrawal symptoms when stopping "cold turkey."

FOOD CHOICES, SERVINGS, AND CARBOHYDRATE COUNTS

GRAINS

Your breakfast menu includes your choice of either one serving of fruit or one serving of grain from the following list:

Food Choice	Serving	Usable Carbohydrates Per Serving	Food Choice	Serving	Usable Carbohydrates Per Serving
Bread (whole grain, 70 calories or less)	1 slice	13	Nutri-Grain (Barley) (Corn)	3/4 cup "	26 27
Cheerios	3/4 cup	12	Nutri-Grain (Rye) (Wheat)	3/4 cup "	25 28
Chex (Bran) (Corn) (Rice) (Wheat)	" " " "	30 19 19 28	Oatmeal (cooked)	1/2 cup	12
Cream of Wheat (cooked)	1/2 cup	13	Post Oat Flakes Post Bran Flakes Product 19	3/4 cup " "	21 23 21
Cream of Rice	"	14	Rice Krispies	3/4 cup	18
Crispix	3/4 cup	19	Shredded Wheat (or Wheat Bran)	"	23
Grapenut Flakes	"	17			
Kashi (Puffed)	"	12	Special K	"	16
Kellogg's 40+ (Bran Flakes)	"	23	Team Flakes Toasties	" "	27 18
Life	"	24	Total (Wheat) (Corn)	" "	17 18
Malt-O-Meal (cooked)	1/2 cup	13	Wheaties	"	18

PROTEIN

Your choice of one serving each at **breakfast, morning snack, lunch, afternoon snack, dinner**, and **evening snack**. Be sure to weigh meat, seafood, and poultry (raw, skinned and boned), with all visible fat removed. Broil, boil, barbecue, microwave, roast, or "fry" in a nonstick pan using Pam spray or an equivalent nonfat, nonstick spray.

Food Choice	Serving	Usable Carbohydrates Per Serving	Food Choice	Serving	Usable Carbohydrates Per Serving
MEAT AND POULTRY			Chicken breast (canned white, water-packed)	2-1/2 oz.	0
Beef heart (ground)	3-1/2 oz.	3			
Beef flank	"	0	Cold cuts (97-98% lean/fat free)	2-1/2 oz.	1
Beef round	"	0	Turkey (white breast)	3-1/2 oz.	0
Chicken breast (fresh or frozen)	"	0	Veal	3-1/2 oz.	0

Food Choice	Serving	Usable Carbohydrates Per Serving
VEGETARIAN		
Tofu	4 oz	2
Veg-e-burger	1/3 cup	3
Veg-e-cutlet or meat substitute	No less than 15 grams of protein per serving	No more than 12 grams of carbohydrate per serving
SEAFOOD		
Catfish	3-1/2 oz.	0
Cod	"	0
Crab	"	1
Haddock	"	0
Halibut	"	0
Lobster	"	1
Orange roughy	"	0
Perch	"	0
Salmon	"	0
Scallops	"	2
Sea Bass	"	0
Shark	"	0
Shrimp	"	1
Snapper	"	0
Sole	"	0
Swordfish	"	0
Trout (Rainbow)	"	0
Tuna (white, fresh or frozen)	"	0
Tuna (canned white albacore, water-packed)	2-1/2 oz.	0
Turbot	3-1/2 oz.	0
DAIRY		
Cheese (fat-free)	2 oz.	0
Cottage cheese (lowfat, plain)	4 oz.	4
Egg (limit if cholesterol is high or use EggBeaters)	1	1
Milk (nonfat)	1 cup	12
Yogurt (nonfat, plain)	1/2 cup	9

"LEAN FOR LIFE" PROTEIN PRODUCTS

Food Choice	Serving	Usable Carbohydrates Per Serving
Protein Bars		
Apple Cinnamon	1 bar	15
Chocolate Delight	"	8
Chocolate Mint	"	13
Double Chocolate	"	13
Honey Almond	"	8
Honey Nougat	"	15
Honey Peanut	"	8
Cinnamon Raisin	"	16
Peanut Butter	"	16
Soups		
Beef and Vegetable	1	5
Cream of Asparagus	"	2
Chicken Boullion	"	1
Creamy Chicken	"	1
Cream of Chicken (with Vegetables)	"	7
Chicken Noodle	"	6
Cream of Mushroom	"	1
Tomato	"	5
Meals		
Madras Curry	1	10
Hearty Beef Stew	"	13
Scrambled Eggs	"	5
Spaghetti Bolognese	"	12
Old Time Chili	"	11
Shakes and Puddings		
Banana Creme Pudding	1	10
Banana Drink/Pudding	"	6
Chocolate Drink/Pudding	"	5
Double Chocolate Pudding	"	9
Rice & Raisin Pudding	"	9
Strawberry Drink/Pudding	"	6
Vanilla Drink/Pudding	"	5
Banana Frosted Shake	1	9
Pina Colada Shake	"	9
Creamy Chocolate Shake	"	7
Creamy Vanilla Shake	"	11
Fruit Drinks		
Orange Drink	"	2
Peach Mango Drink	"	2
Pineapple-Apricot Drink	"	3
Pink Grapefruit Drink	"	2
Wildberry Drink	"	3
Hot Drinks		
Cafe Amaretto	1	5
Cafe Au Lait	"	5
Cappuccino	"	4
Creamy Hot Cocoa	"	5
Hot Chocolate	"	4
Irish Creme Hot Cocoa	"	5

Product availability is subject to change. Some may require special order.

VEGETABLES

Your choice of one serving each at *lunch* and *dinner*. Measure raw, frozen (thawed), water packed (drained), unless otherwise stated. No sugar added.

Food Choice	Serving	Usable Carbohydrates Per Serving	Food Choice	Serving	Usable Carbohydrates Per Serving
Asparagus	1 cup	8	Mushrooms, raw	2 cups	7
Bean sprouts	"	14	Okra	1 cup	8
Broccoli	"	5	Onion	1/2 cup	6
Cabbage	"	4	Pepper	1 small	4
Carrots	1/2 cup	8	(red or green)		
Celery	1 cup	6	Spinach (raw)	2 cups	4
Chinese pea pods	"	11	(cooked)	1 cup	7
Cauliflower	"	5	String beans	"	8
Collard greens	1 cup	8	Sauerkraut	"	10
Cucumbers	"	3	Tomato	1 small	5
Jicama	1/2 cup	5	Zucchini	1 cup	4

FRUITS

Your choice of one serving each at *breakfast* (when not choosing a grain), *lunch* and *dinner*. Be sure your daily fruit choices include at least one citrus (indicated with a *). Choose fresh, frozen (thawed), or water packed (without sugar or fruit juice).

Food Choice	Serving	Usable Carbohydrates Per Serving	Food Choice	Serving	Usable Carbohydrates Per Serving
Apple	1, 2-1/2" dia.	17	Honeydew melon	1/6 (6-1/2" dia)	20
Applesauce	1/2 cup	14	Orange*	1 small	14
(unsweetened)			Orange juice*	4 oz.	12
Apricots (fresh)	2 medium	9	(unsweetened)		
(dried)	4 halves	9	Papaya	1/2 cup, cubed	7
Banana	1/2 small	13	Peach	1 small	10
Blackberries	2/3 cup	12	Pear (Bartlett)	1/2 small	13
Blueberries	"	14	Persimmon	1	8
Boysenberries	"	11	Pineapple	1/2 cup, cubed	10
Casaba melon	1/4 (6-1/2" dia.)	4	Raisins	1/2 oz.	11
Cantaloupe	1/4 (6" dia.)	11	Raspberries	2/3 cup	10
Cherries	10	11	Rhubarb	1 cup	7
Dates	2	13	Strawberries	1 cup	11
Grapefruit*	1/2 small	10	Tangerine*	1 (2-1/2" dia.)	9
Grapefruit juice*	4 oz.	11	Watermelon	1/2 cup, cubed	6

MISCELLANEOUS

Your choice of one serving, twice per day, with the meals of your choice.

Food Choice	Serving	Usable Carbohydrates Per Serving	Food Choice	Serving	Usable Carbohydrates Per Serving
Gelatin (diet)	1/2 cup	0	Mustard	1 tsp.	0
Green onion (tops)	1 tsp.	0	Peppers, jalapeño	2 small	2
Horseradish	"	1	Pimento	"	1
Margarine	1 Tbs.	0	Radishes	2 medium	1
(nonfat, 5 cal max.)			Vinegar (unseasoned)	2 Tbs.	2

WHAT ARE LEAN FOR LIFE PROTEIN PRODUCTS?

In addition to the many food choices included in the Protein section of your "Phase I: Weight Loss" menu, you will find a listing that features dozens of Lean for Life protein snacks and products. These products have been designed specifically for use on the weight-loss program and as a delicious, healthy, convenient snack or meal replacement.

While it's entirely realistic for you to succeed on the program without using *any* of the specific products mentioned in this book, they can enhance your experience by providing more of what this program is all about: choices.

The Lean for Life product line offers dozens of options—everything from chewy Chocolate Mint and Cinnamon Oatmeal Raisin Snack Bars to Home Style Chicken Noodle Soup to Hearty Beef Stew. Choices include Banana Cream Pudding and Double Chocolate Pudding, and there are more than a dozen beverages available—everything from Peach-Mango Fruit Drink, Vanilla and Pina Colada Shakes to Hot Chocolate and Cafe Amaretto.

Keep in mind that the Lean for Life line of protein supplements and food products is ever-changing. Formulas are constantly being improved and new products are regularly introduced. Updated product lists are always available upon request. To find out what's new—or to order a sampler pack containing a selection of the most popular items—see the Resources section of this book.

VITAMIN AND MINERAL SUPPLEMENTS

Vitamins are an essential part of the Lean for Life program. They help maximize absorption and utilization of the food you eat, as well as safeguard against nutritional deficiencies.

During "Phase 1: Weight Loss," you will be taking two multiple vitamin and mineral supplements, three times a day, with meals. Lean for Life vitamins have been developed for use with the program. The required vitamins and minerals are present in optimal strengths and the minerals have been chelated for easier assimilation. Available in our clinics to Lindora patients, Lean for Life vitamin-with-mineral supplements may be ordered by mail and phone. See the Resources section of this book for more information.

If you prefer to use an equivalent high-quality multiple vitamin with mineral supplement, carefully compare the label with this ingredient list.

		%USRDA*
Vitamin A (Acetate)	5000IU	100%
Vitamin D (Ergocalciferol)	400IU	100%
Vitamin E (d-Alpha Tocopheryl Acetate)	200IU	667%
Vitamin C (Ascorbic Acid)	600mg	1000%
Folic Acid	400mcg	100%
Vitamin B-1 (Thiamine HCl)	100mg	6667%
Vitamin B-2 (Riboflavin)	100mg	5882%
Niacinamide	100mg	500%
Vitamin B-6 (Pyridoxine)	100mg	5000%
Vitamin B-12 (Cyanocobalamin)	500mcg	8333%
Biofin	100mcg	33%
Pantothenic Acid (d-Calcium Pantothenate)	100mg	1000%
Calcium (Carbonate Di-Calcium Phosphate)	400mg	40%
Phosphorous (Di-Calcium Phosphate)	100mg	10%
Iodine (Kelp)	100mcg	67%
Iron (Gluconate)	15mg	83%
Magnesium (Oxide)	200mg	50%
Copper (Gluconate)	2mg	100%
Zinc (Gluconate)	40mg	267%
Potassium (Gluconate)	99mg	**
Manganese (Gluconate)	5mg	**
Chromium (Yeast)	10mcg	**
Rutin	50mg	***
Lemon Bioflavinoids Complex	200mg	***
Inositol	400mg	***
Choline (Bitartrate)	700mg	**
Para Amino Benzoic Acid	100mg	***

*Percentage of U.S. Recommended Daily Allowance.
**Percentage of U.S. Recommended Daily Allowance Not Established.
***Need in human nutrition not established.

Some people experience an aftertaste when taking vitamins. If you're one of them, you might want to try these simple remedies:

1. Take your vitamins halfway through your meal and then finish eating.

2. Freeze your vitamins. This allows them to be absorbed more slowly, which seems to enhance tolerance in people who are sensitive to vitamin and mineral supplements.

POTASSIUM AND SODIUM

While most people get the potassium they need—50 to 100 milliequivalents (mEq) per day—from the foods they eat, there are occasions when one may need extra potassium. People being treated with diuretics for high blood pressure, for example, are typically advised to take potassium supplements to replace potassium lost in the urine. Similarly, the body can lose large amounts of potassium any time there is a large flow of urine, as may happen when a person is in ketosis and is drinking a lot of fluids.

A day's supply of the vitamin and mineral supplements developed for use by Lindora patients contains potassium, as do some of the Lean for Life protein supplements. The amount may not be adequate for all individuals, so additional supplementation may be required.

If your blood potassium level is low, it's wise to take enough potassium to raise and maintain it in the mid-normal to high-normal range. Symptoms such as muscle weakness and/or muscle cramps are strongly suggestive of a potassium deficiency, and merit prompt attention to prevent further depletion and such potentially serious consequences as irregularities in heart rhythm.

Like potassium, sodium is present in the foods we eat, usually in adequate amounts to meet ordinary demands. Normal sodium intake is usually enough to maintain an adequate amount of liquid in our blood vessels, and thus to maintain a normal blood pressure.

The total amount of liquid within the blood vessels decreases, however, when people are on a low-carbohydrate weight-loss program. As a result, blood pressure can drop when a person stands suddenly from a seated or horizontal position, causing weakness, lightheadedness, and dizziness. This is called orthostatic hypotension (low blood pressure resulting from a change in position).

To prevent this, we encourage our patients to add salt to their food during the weight loss phase. The resulting restoration of normal blood volume sometimes results in a temporary weight increase, but any such gain is soon reversed as weight loss proceeds.

It's prudent to monitor your blood pressure during the first week of the program, especially if you experience any of the symptoms described.

Potassium is available over the counter. However, your need for potassium and/or sodium supplementation can best be determined by consulting your physician or health-care professional. This is absolutely essential if you are taking medication regularly or being treated for a chronic disease. Your physician can obtain additional information about this and all other aspects of the Lean for Life program by telephoning the medical consultation number featured in the Resources section of this book.

ANY QUESTIONS?

Q: *Can anyone do a ketogenic program?*

A: While ketosis is a normal part of the body's fat-burning metabolism, there are some people for whom a ketogenic program is not recommended:

- ❑   women who are pregnant or nursing
- ❑   those with serious liver or kidney diseases
- ❑   Type 1, insulin-dependent diabetics

If you have any concerns or questions, be sure to consult with your health-care professional before beginning this program.

ACTION PLANNING

*You will know, day by day, exactly
what is working for you*

"People are always blaming their circumstances for what they are," observed Irish author and playwright George Bernard Shaw. "I don't believe in circumstances."

Shaw clearly had little patience for those who wallowed in inertia and indecision. He would have loved the Lean for Life program.

"The people who get on in this world," he observed, "are the people who get up and look for the circumstances they want, and if they can't find them, *make* them."

That's exactly what your Daily Action Plan supports you in doing: creating "circumstances" in which you can enhance your success by stacking the deck in your favor.

The Daily Action Plan is a simple, easy-to-keep record you'll complete every day while on the program. To make it convenient for you, a Daily Action Plan is included for each day of the program. As you get into the habit of maintaining your Daily Action Plan, you'll notice it provides insights and information that will help you stay focused and motivated.

Lean *for* Life®
DAILY ACTION PLAN

Week _Ⓐ2_ Day _11_ Date _3/5_

Time	Meal Plans	Serving Size	Carbs (grams)
7:00 A.M.	**Breakfast** Ⓑ		Ⓒ
	Protein _EGG_	1	1
	Fruit or grain _WHEAT BREAD_	1 SLICE	13
	Beverage _DECAF COFFEE_	8 OZ	θ
	+ WATER ↓	8 OZ	θ
	WATER	30 OZ	θ
10:30 A.M.	**Snack** _FAT-FREE CHEESE_	2 OZ	θ
12:30 P.M.	**Lunch**		
	Protein _CANNED TUNA_	2½ OZ	θ
	Vegetable _TOMATO_	1 SMALL	5
	Lettuce + TBSP DRESSING	2 CUPS	3
	Fruit _STRAWBERRIES_	1 CUP	11
	Beverage _WATER_	18 OZ	θ
	Miscellaneous _RADISHES_	2	1
	WATER	30 OZ	θ
3:30 P.M	**Snack** _HONEY PEANUT PROTEIN BAR_	1	8
6:15 P.M.	**Dinner**		
	Protein _CHICKEN BREAST_	3½ OZ	θ
	Vegetable _ASPARAGUS_	1 CUP	8
	Lettuce + 1 TBSP DRESSING	2 CUPS	2
	Fruit _UNSW. APPLESAUCE_	½ CUP	14
	Beverage _HERB TEA +_	10 OZ	θ
	Miscellaneous _WATER_	8 OZ	θ
	DIET GELATIN	½ CUP	θ
8:45 P.M	**Snack** _NON-FAT MILK_	1 CUP	12
		TOTAL	78 Ⓓ

Keto Reading Ⓔ MODERATE
Weight Ⓕ 167
Vitamins 2 AM Ⓖ 2 Noon   2 PM
Water Ⓗ 16, 30, 18, 30, 10, 8 = 112 OZ
Activities Ⓘ 30 MINUTE WALK
  20 LEG LIFTS
  TOOK STAIRS TO WORK

Pedometer Steps Ⓙ 7,554

BODY MEASUREMENTS Ⓚ

Chest 38½		Hips 43	
Waist 31¼		Thighs 25¼	
Abdomen 38			

SUCCESS LEARNING TOOLS Ⓛ

Read pages # 108 - 114
Audio Tapes RELAXATION
Video
CD-ROM
Affirmation Ⓜ I CREATE MY OWN JOY!
  I LOVE TO EXERCISE!
  I AM LEAN + HEALTHY!

Other READ MOTIVATOR CARD BEFORE
Plan to Overcome Today's Obstacles: SLEEP
  Ⓝ
TAKE PROTEIN BAR TO EAT DURING
AFTERNOON MEETING. AVOID
SWEET ROLL TRAY! DRINK 30 OZ
WATER DURING MEETING.
Notes:
CALL DEBBIE TO ASK ABOUT
FRIDAY'S MENU. REQUEST
GRILLED CHICKEN, RAW VEGGIES,
FRUIT AND LETTUCE.

STAY FOCUSED — IT'S WORKING!

Let's take a line-by-line look at a sample Daily Action Plan sheet completed by Stephanie, who lost 62 pounds on the program.

A. Begin by filling out the date, week, and day of your program. Remember that "Phase 1: Weight Loss" lasts up to 28 days, unless you are under medical supervision, in which case the length of your program will be determined by you and the medical staff.

B. Write down *everything* you eat and drink, *every time* you eat or drink. Many well-intentioned people are oblivious to what—and how much—they consume. Before every meal or snack, jot down the time, what you're eating, and how much.

C. During "Phase 1: Weight Loss," you will also keep track of how many grams of carbohydrates you're eating. *Before you eat anything during this phase, know how many carbohydrates it contains.*

D. At the end of the day, add up your total carbohydrate intake.

E. Check your ketone measuring strip or "ketostick" every morning, 15 seconds after passing it through your urine stream. Record the result. If on any morning during the weight-loss phase your ketostick doesn't show color, carefully review the previous day's Action Plan. Look for clues as to what bumped you out of ketosis. Check the number of carbohydrates you ate the previous day. If you take in too many carbs, you will go out of ketosis. Don't beat

WHY WEIGH?

Does the idea of stepping on the scale send shivers down your spine? For some, weighing themselves ranks right up there with oral surgery, public speaking, and unexpected letters from the IRS.

But rather than thinking of the scale as judge and jury or some measure of your value as a person, remember what it really measures: how much your body weighs. It's a resource that provides valuable information you can't get any other way. It's a tool—nothing more, nothing less.

Just as an architect wouldn't think of designing a house before measuring the lot, why do a weight-loss program without measuring your progress along the way?

yourself up, but instead learn from your mistakes so you don't repeat them. Carefully monitor how many carbohydrates you consume.

F. Weigh yourself every morning, ideally around the same time every day. Whenever possible, weigh the same way every day, nude and after emptying your bladder. Record your weight.

G. Be sure to take your Lean for Life vitamins and mineral supplements (or an equivalent). During "Phase 1: Weight Loss," take two with *each meal* and check it off on your Action Plan. During "Phase 2: Metabolic Adjustment" and "Phase 3: Lifetime Maintenance," you'll be taking fewer vitamin and mineral tablets because you'll be eating more.

H. During "Phase 1: Weight Loss," it's essential that you drink a minimum of 80 ounces of water or other calorie-free beverages every day. Water is preferable. Keep track of everything you drink and log it in.

I. Write down the exercise you do throughout the day.

J. When you start using a pedometer (step counter), which we'll discuss later, you'll be able to keep a record of the number of steps you've walked each day. Exercise and activity provide countless physical and psychological payoffs: they elevate your mood, boost your metabolism, improve your ability to burn fat for fuel,

Another Lean for Life Sucess Story

"When I began the program, I focused on the 43 pounds I wanted to lose. It never occurred to me that what I might gain would turn out to be every bit as meaningful. The strategies and skills I learned have enhanced my health, my relationships, and my work. I no longer see my future as something that will happen to me. I now realize that the choices I make—or don't make—today directly affect the quality of my life tomorrow."

— Laura

accelerate weight loss, tone and firm your body, and help you feel more relaxed and less hungry.

K. Refer to the "Measure Up" box on page 21.

L. You will be instructed on these aspects of the program throughout the book.

M. Every day, you'll want to write down one or two statements that you will repeat to yourself throughout the day. Begin these statements with the words "I am...", and fill in the blank by describing what you are ready to experience that day. For example, "I am enjoying my Lean for Life program," or "I am doing something that matters to me!" As you'll soon discover, these affirmations and the other mental training activities you'll be learning will become powerful tools to help you become lean and healthy.

N. Anticipate challenges. First thing every morning, review your schedule and consider any obstacles you expect to encounter during your day. What is your plan of action for overcoming that particular challenge? Write it down. Remember your plan and be ready to implement it.

As you begin using your Daily Action Plan, you'll notice certain patterns emerging. Many of these patterns will be positive, but others will not. The beauty of keeping a Daily Action Plan is that it provides you a wealth of information about what's working and what isn't.

Knowledge is power. Your Daily Action Plan is a powerful resource that will help you stay aware and focused on achieving your goal.

TODAY IS YOUR FIRST "PROTEIN DAY"

"Phase 1: Weight Loss" begins with a maximum of three Protein Days. Today will be your first. During your Protein Days, you'll be eating approximately 100 grams of protein a day, while keeping your carbohydrate intake low—somewhere in the neighborhood of 50 grams. This ensures that you will begin burning fat as rapidly as possible.

What distinguishes these first days from the rest of "Phase 1: Weight Loss" is that you will be eating only protein-based foods—no fruits, vegetables, or other foods during this time. You may eat high-protein, low-carbohydrate foods such as egg whites, tuna, turkey or chicken breast, low-fat tofu, and other foods from the Protein list found on pages 32–33. Throughout the program—but especially during the Protein Days—many Lindora patients enjoy the convenience and

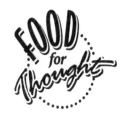

"It's a funny thing about life; if you refuse to accept anything but the best, you very often get it."

— W. Somerset Maugham

Lean *for* Life®
DAILY ACTION PLAN

PROTEIN DAY

Week ___I___ Day ___I___ Date _____

Time	Meal Plans	Serving Size	Carbs (grams)
	Breakfast		
	Protein		
	Beverage		
	Protein Snack		
	Lunch		
	Protein		
	Beverage		
	Protein Snack		
	Dinner		
	Protein		
	Beverage		
	Protein Snack		
		TOTAL	

Keto Reading _____

Weight _____

Vitamins   AM   Noon   PM

Water _____

Activities _____
_____
_____

Pedometer Steps _____

WEEKLY BODY MEASUREMENTS

Chest _____ Hips _____

Waist _____ Thighs _____

Abdomen _____

SUCCESS LEARNING TOOLS

Read pages # _____

Audio Tape _____

Video _____

CD-ROM _____

Bio-Card™ _____

Affirmation _____

Other _____

Plan to Overcome Today's Obstacles:
_____
_____
_____
_____

Notes:
_____
_____
_____
_____

**TODAY IS YOUR FIRST PROTEIN DAY
UNLESS OTHERWISE DIRECTED
BY YOUR HEALTH CARE PROFESSIONAL.**

variety of eating delicious, high-quality medical-grade Lean for Life high protein nutritional products. (See the Resources section for more information.) By mixing and matching your food and protein product choices, you can enjoy a wide variety of tastes during your Protein Days.

HOW TO DO YOUR PROTEIN DAYS

❑ Eat at least six (6) protein servings a day (one each for breakfast, morning snack, lunch, afternoon snack, dinner, and evening snack). Choose foods from the "Phase 1: Weight Loss" Protein list and/or Lean for Life protein products. Each selection equals one serving. Depending on your current weight and level of activity, you may need more than six to control your hunger and maintain your energy. Let your ketostick reading and how you're feeling be your guide. Never have fewer than six servings per day—you need the protein!

❑ Use your Daily Action Plan to write down each protein serving you eat and how many carbohydrate grams it contains. Aim for a daily total of approximately 50 to 100 grams of carbohydrates.

❑ Take two Lean for Life vitamin/mineral supplements, or an equivalent, three times a day, with meals.

❑ Drink at least 80 ounces of water or other calorie-free beverages a day.

❑ Unless you have high blood pressure, you may add salt to your food during your Protein Days. If you tend to have lower blood pressure, the addition of salt may help alleviate the slight dizziness some dieters occasionally experience.

❑ On the morning of your second Protein Day, empty your bladder and then test your urine with a ketostick to determine whether you're in ketosis. If your ketostick shows a pink to purple color, you are in ketosis and can immediately begin the "Phase 1: Weight Loss" menu plan. Most people find it takes three full Protein Days to achieve "good color," so don't be discouraged. After a maximum of three Protein Days, move on to the weight-loss menu plan regardless of the color on your ketostick (unless you are under medical supervision). You will continue testing for ketosis every morning throughout "Phase 1: Weight Loss."

"WHAT SHOULD I EAT ON MY PROTEIN DAYS?"

The choice is yours. With the variety of options available, you can enjoy a different menu on every one of your Protein Days. **Choose from the protein servings on pages 32 and 33.** Here's a sample menu:

BREAKFAST
2 scrambled egg whites OR
Lean for Life Cafe Au Lait Vanilla

MORNING SNACK
2 ounces of fat-free cheese OR
I Lean for Life Creamy Hot Cocoa

LUNCH
2 1/2 ounces, water-packed tuna OR
I Lean for Life Homestyle Chicken Soup with Noodles

AFTERNOON SNACK
4 ounces low-fat cottage cheese OR
I Lean for Life Peanut Butter Bar

DINNER
3 1/2 ounces chicken or turkey breast OR
I Lean for Life Savory Beef Soup with Vegetables

EVENING SNACK
2 1/2 ounces lean/fat-free cold cuts OR
I Lean for Life Pina Colada Frosted Shake

HOW WILL I FEEL WHILE ON THE PROGRAM?

It's a question that's asked every day in our clinics. The answer varies as much as the people who ask it. Many people feel terrific from the very first day. They marvel at the fact they're not hungry, and comment on their increased energy and overall sense of well-being.

Others, however, find the process more challenging, occasionally experiencing *temporary food withdrawal symptoms*. If this happens to you, don't be alarmed. It's perfectly normal for your body to react whenever you make significant changes in the way you eat. I tell you this not because you *will* experience any symptoms or side effects, but because it's possible that you *may*.

These reactions may include mild or brief episodes of constipation, diarrhea, heartburn, nausea, indigestion, fluid retention and headaches.

Some people also experience brief bouts of fatigue, insomnia, depression, and/or irritability.

One of the consequences of carbohydrate depletion and ketosis is a reduction of body water. This can result in a lowering of blood pressure. For people who normally have high blood pressure, this is an added benefit. In fact, if you are taking medication for high blood pressure, talk with your doctor. You may find that over time, it's possible to reduce your dosage.

If your blood pressure tends to be normal or lower than normal, it's possible that you may experience lightheadedness and dizziness, especially when standing up quickly. If this happens, don't panic. Stand more slowly and allow your body to adjust. You may want to monitor your blood pressure. In any event, *it's essential to drink plenty of fluids and make sure you're getting enough salt in your diet*. You can do this by adding table salt to your food and by drinking chicken bouillon.

ANY QUESTIONS?

Q: *Eighty ounces of water? I'll float away! Why is drinking that much water so important?*

A. Water cleanses your system, curbs appetite, reduces fluid retention, and relieves constipation. It also flushes out the toxic chemicals, such as organophosphates used in agriculture, that have been stored in fat and released into the bloodstream as the fat is being used.

Q: *Can I use packaged protein supplements from the grocery store?*

A: No, because most contain too many carbohydrates and not enough protein. Patients on the program use specially formulated, medical-grade supplements that are high in protein and contain limited carbohydrates.

DAY
2

THE SELF-SABOTAGE SHUFFLE

You will learn through awareness and action how to stop sabotaging yourself.

Congratulations. You're doing it! You're now beginning the second of your three Protein Days. Although it's unlikely you're already in ketosis, you may have started to notice that something different is happening to your body. You may have awakened this morning "feeling thinner," and there may be other ways in which you feel different physically. If you have any discomfort, know that it's only temporary. You may want to review the section titled "How Will I Feel While on the Program?" from yesterday.

As you begin moving down this path you've chosen, now is the perfect time to take a look at some of the detours that might slow you down.

Most weight-loss and self-improvement programs steer clear of addressing physical and psychological obstacles. At Lindora, however, we've learned from experience that the best way to turn obstacles into opportunities is to anticipate them and to develop strategies for overcoming them.

During the course of your program, any number of things could go wrong. You can't plan for the fender bender that could happen on your way home from work any more than you can control the random earthquake, flood, or hurricane that might temporarily disrupt your life. But since they're not under your control anyway, let's put these kinds of catastrophes into a box, label it "Uncontrollable Life Events," and store it out of sight and out of mind for now.

Let's focus instead on what you *can* control: what you put into your mouth every day. People often define this control too narrowly. They say things like: "Today's a lost cause—I've got a business meeting at an Italian restaurant," or "How am I supposed to eat on the program when I'm hosting a pizza party for my daughter's Girl Scout troop?"

There's no question that some challenges are tougher than others. Whenever possible, it's best to steer clear of potential problem situations during the weight-loss phase of your program. If they're truly unavoidable, the task then becomes how to successfully navigate those choppy waters of temptation.

Each of us is ultimately responsible for our own actions. You have the ability to deal with the inevitable inconveniences and difficulties that are sure to occur while doing a program in which you're eating differently from the way you usually do.

The key word here is *differently*. Most of us find it tough to change our patterns and do things differently. Change isn't easy. Routines become a way of life. When we know what to expect, we don't have to think about it.

Attempts at change are most always met with some inner resistance. Sometimes, it's obvious when this is happening. Comments like "I'm tired of this—I want something else" or "I'm not walking in this weather. Those clouds are going to break loose any minute!" are sure signs you're struggling with the part of yourself that's determined to maintain the status quo.

Steve, a Lindora patient who lost 34 pounds in eight weeks, caught himself complaining one day that it just "wasn't fair" that he wouldn't be able to "pig out" at his softball league's year-end barbecue bash. Mid-sentence, Steve couldn't help but laugh. "Wow! I sound exactly like my 2-year-old when she throws a tantrum," he observed. "The only difference is that I don't hold my breath!"

Resistance isn't always verbalized. In fact, it often surfaces in more subtle ways. Here are just a few examples, shared by four Lindora patients:

"I went grocery shopping the other night without a list. I was also hungry, which only made matters worse. As I was unpacking the groceries, my husband came home and noticed a bag of chocolate cookies. If they weren't my favorite kind, I'd swear someone put them in my basket by mistake. I don't even remember taking them off the shelf."

— Judy

Lean *for* Life®
DAILY ACTION PLAN

PROTEIN DAY

Week ___1___ Day ___2___ Date _____

Time	Meal Plans	Serving Size	Carbs (grams)
____	**Breakfast**		
	Protein		
	Beverage		
____	**Protein Snack**		
____	**Lunch**		
	Protein		
	Beverage		
____	**Protein Snack**		
____	**Dinner**		
	Protein		
	Beverage		
____	**Protein Snack**		
		TOTAL	

Keto Reading _____
Weight _____
Vitamins   AM   Noon   PM
Water _____

Activities _____

\# Pedometer Steps _____

WEEKLY BODY MEASUREMENTS
Chest _____ Hips _____
Waist _____ Thighs _____
Abdomen _____

SUCCESS LEARNING TOOLS
Read pages # _____
Audio Tape _____
Video _____
CD-ROM _____
Bio-Card™ _____
Affirmation _____

Other _____
Plan to Overcome Today's Obstacles: _____

Notes: _____

TODAY IS YOUR SECOND PROTEIN DAY
UNLESS OTHERWISE DIRECTED
BY YOUR HEALTH CARE PROFESSIONAL.

"I was making dinner for the kids last night, and before I knew it, I'd nibbled a whole hamburger bun. After I realized it, I just stood there thinking, 'How—and why—did *that* happen?'"

— John

"All day, I was looking forward to walking after work. It's been really chilly, just how I like it. But then my friends Viki and Patricia called. They were heading to the mall to check out a big sale on linens. I needed new bedding, so I met them there. I got a terrific deal on pillow cases, but I never did take my walk."

— Cassie

"I guess I should know better than to talk on the phone while I'm making dinner. Gary called to tell me about the committee meeting I missed last week. I was paying more attention to what he had to say than to my food. I didn't realize it until later when I was cleaning up, but I nearly doubled my serving sizes."

— Christopher

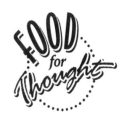

"Whether you think you can or think you can't, you're right."

—Henry Ford

Four different people facing four different challenges. Each had the opportunity to control the situation, yet sabotaged him- or herself by not thinking, not planning, and not being fully aware. Instead of evaluating the situation and making a choice that reflected their goal, each went temporarily blank. The result? In each case, the old habits re-emerged.

Whenever we ask people who are sabotaging themselves what they want to achieve, they inevitably insist that they want to lose weight. They want to become Lean for Life. So then why don't they "just do it"? If only it were that easy! No matter how committed a *part* of you is to losing weight, there's *another* part that is inevitably going to resist change. That's the voice that says, "C'mon, one little piece won't kill you" or "You deserve it—you've been good!"

On Day 12, you'll learn all about your personal "Inner Committee" and how you can decide which voice will wield the greatest influence. For now, it's important to understand that change requires a heightened

TODAY'S EATING PLAN

Q: *What's my meal plan for today?*

A: Is your ketostick showing color yet? After just one full Protein Day, it's unlikely, but checking it is an important habit to develop. Continue following your Protein Day eating plan. And while you're at it, take a walk!

DO YOU HAVE "BODY IMAGE DEPRESSION?"

Do you think about the shape, strength, and/or size of your body on a daily basis? Do you wish you looked significantly different from the way you do today? Do you feel fat, no matter how much weight you lose or how much positive feedback you receive? Are you jealous of, or intimidated by, those you consider more attractive and fit? Do you often feel unattractive or self-conscious no matter what you wear? Do you ever attempt to hide your body from your intimate partner or avoid looking at yourself in the mirror?

These are just a few of the warning signs of "Body Image Depression," which clinical psychologist Ellen McGrath defines in her groundbreaking book, *When Feeling Bad Is Good* (Bantam Books, 1994), as "the negative feelings of shame, contempt, and disappointment in our bodies" that many of us—especially women—experience "as we attempt to live up to impossible cultural standards of physical perfection, beauty, sex appeal, youth, and fashion."

Women, McGrath suggests, are especially vulnerable to Body Image Depression. "We are conditioned from infancy to believe that the major source of our worth is how attractive we are to others, especially men," McGrath writes. "A disproportionate premium is placed on being beautiful, pretty, attractive, cute, and sexy... For a vast majority of women, beauty remains the primary currency of our value and worth."

The pressure to be physically perfect and remain forever young, McGrath believes, are two of the most consistent sources of depression among women.

"The depressing reality is that the cultural pressures for female perfection are so strong and pervasive that even if we resist or reject them, they still continue to haunt most of us."

In her book, McGrath offers a series of "Action Strategies" for overcoming Body Image Depression.

"It's important to see yourself as a problem-solver rather than a victim," McGrath says. "Get active. Create your own definition of what's healthy and attractive. Talk with other women about how cultural standards have changed in recent years. Make a list of the women you most admire—it can be a liberating reminder that many of the world's most accomplished women are valued and respected more for their character, courage, and substance rather than for their degree of 'physical perfection.'"

state of awareness of what you are doing. Pay close attention to your thoughts and actions by making a conscious effort to be aware.

By taking a close look at your self-sabotage strategies as they occur, you're bound to discover patterns. Do you slip more at the end of the day when you're tired? Are your defenses down when you're stressed, angry, or on deadline? Do you tend to lose your focus on weekends?

Recognizing these patterns will help you become more aware of your personal blind spots. Is there a way to pace yourself or build exercise into your day so that you don't feel so vulnerable at dinnertime? Can you come up with other ways of reacting to stress or anger? Can you structure your weekends so they're no longer a 48-hour excuse for "blowing it"?

This is a program that can do more than change your body. It can also change your life. In the process of changing your eating and exercise habits, you will discover things about yourself you never knew before. The self-awareness you'll gain during the coming weeks can serve you in every area of your life. By the time you've completed this program, you'll not only be leaner and healthier, you'll be better prepared than ever to turn obstacles into opportunities.

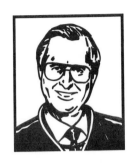

DR. STAMPER

"Motivation is a decision. Remind yourself several times every day why you've decided to become Lean for Life."

THE LANGUAGE OF SELF-SABOTAGE

Do you know who tells you the most important words you'll ever hear? You do. That little voice within your head, the one that talks to you hundreds of times every day, is an incredibly influential character.

What voice, you ask? You say you don't have one?

Another Lean for Life Success Story

"I've come to realize that the actions I take create the results I get. Someone once commented that the harder he worked, the luckier he got. It's true. If I really want something, I do everything within my power to make it happen. When I'm truly committed, no temptation is strong enough to get in my way. It's not always easy, but everything has a price. If this simple truth were as easy to swallow as pizza or pistachios, I wouldn't have spent the past 20 years wishing I weighed 20 pounds less."

—Rick

THEN&NOW

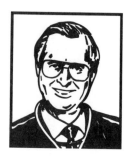

DR. STAMPER

"Losing weight—
and keeping it off—
has at least
as much to do
with what we put
in our minds as
what we put
in our mouths."

That's the voice I'm talking about! Your inner voice—the one that says, "Turn left at the next light" or "You forgot to give Mom a call"—has considerable impact on the way you live. While your inner voice generally does its best to help and protect you ("You'd better drive slower in this rain"), it's not a big fan of change. In fact, it can be downright stubborn.

Let's look at five of the most common self-sabotage patterns people fall into and the negative self-talk, or inner dialogue, that fuels them.

All or Nothing Thinkers tend to see the world in black and white. If their performance falls short of their expectations, they see themselves as failures. Kate, for example, lost 23 pounds on the program, but couldn't take pride in her accomplishment. Why? Because her goal was to lose 25 and she kept telling herself that she "would never make it."

Overgeneralizers zero in on a single negative event or experience as proof of failure. Three weeks into his program, when Adam hit a temporary plateau where he didn't lose any weight, his first inclination was to give up: "I *told* you it wouldn't work. I may as well quit right now!"

Labelers can be brutal, especially with themselves. When Heidi gained two pounds the week after being laid off from a job she loved, her assessment of the situation was especially harsh: "I'm a total loser. I'm unemployed and I'm fat!"

Doom-and-Gloomers discount their success by insisting that, for whatever reason, their achievements "don't count." They hold on to negative beliefs, even when they've been contradicted by positive experiences. When Rebecca achieved her goal of losing 45 pounds, she had trouble enjoying her achievement. Her first reaction: "I don't really see that much difference. And who knows if it'll stay off, anyway? Only time will tell."

Conclusion Jumpers make general statements that have no basis in fact. Gustavo was enthusiastic about beginning the program until he learned that activity was an essential part of the overall strategy. "I can't walk," he announced. "Walking cramps my legs up." When one of our clinic nurses asked when he last experienced leg cramps, Gustavo admitted he never had, but quickly added that he was "positive" he would. By jumping to this conclusion, he overlooked the obvious: that the 70 extra pounds he had been carrying for the past six years were much more punishing on his legs than a daily walk.

Later in the program, we'll discuss how you can change this kind of negative inner dialogue. But until you realize a problem exists, it's tough to overcome it. Over the next several days, make a point to listen to the messages you convey to yourself through words and thoughts. How often—and how easily—do you fall into these patterns? By recognizing these traps, you'll be less likely to fall victim to them in the future.

GENTLE EXERCISE AND THE MAGICAL MITOCHONDRIA

*You can exercise more gently than you
thought and still lose fat.*

Did you know you can burn fat by exercising *gently*? Many people still believe that for exercise to make a difference, it has to be exhausting. For years, "No Pain, No Gain" was the anthem of the active. We were led to believe that unless our hearts were racing, our breath was short, and we ended our workout drenched, we had somehow shortchanged ourselves.

WHEN LESS IS MORE

In fact, the opposite is true. Doctors, health researchers, and fitness experts now know that a consistent program of moderate exercise is ultimately the safest, most effective approach for achieving and maintaining good health.

In March 1993, an expert panel was assembled by the American College of Sports Medicine and the U.S. Centers for Disease Control and Prevention, in conjunction with the President's Council on Physical Fitness and Sports. Concluding that only 22% of American adults are getting enough exercise, the panel speculated that "previous public health efforts to promote

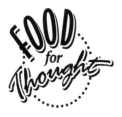

health efforts to promote physical activity have overemphasized the importance of high-intensity exercise."

Gentle exercise, such as walking, is now the accepted approach in exercise and fitness training. What qualifies as "gentle"? Any continuous movement of your hips and knees that you do without becoming breathless. If, while exercising, you can't talk without feeling short of breath, slow down: it's not gentle enough.

In addition to being easier to do and less likely to cause injury than more vigorous exercise, gentle exercise has been proven to be the most effective way to increase the amount of mitochondria in your body.

MITO-WHAT?

Mitochondria. They're the tiny, egg-shaped structures in your cells that serve as fat-burning furnaces. Too small to be seen with an ordinary microscope, there are trillions in every human body. The more mitochondrial surface you have in your cells, the easier it is for your body to burn stored fat for fuel. If you want to burn more body fat, you need to increase the mitochondrial surface in your cells.

How can you do this? By increasing the amount of gentle exercise you do every day, you will increase the mitochondria in your muscle cells. The result? It'll be easier for your body to burn stored fat for fuel.

Increased amount of gentle exercise ➡ Increased amount of mitochondrial surface ➡ Increased ability to use stored fat for fuel

MEET MR. MITO

At Lindora, we encourage our patients to become "Mitochondriacs." We even developed a mascot to help remind them that movement matters. We call him "Mr. Mito." You've already seen his picture on your Daily Action Plan, and you'll be seeing more of him in the coming weeks. Think of him as your personal exercise and activity coach. He'll help you increase your daily activity level by reminding you to "Step It Up!" and showing you how to "exercise" without having to find an extra hour in your busy day. He'll have plenty of tips to share with you throughout the book.

Another Lean for Life Success Story

*"I remember when I first received my pedometer and was
encouraged to walk at least 10,000 steps a day. I thought
to myself, 'Yeah, right!' I could barely walk to the
bathroom. For the first few months, I only logged
about 2,000 steps a day. But as my weight
dropped, I've been able to walk more. I'm down
120 pounds and I often do 10,000 steps in a day."*

THEN&NOW

— *Marsha*

HOW MUCH GENTLE EXERCISE DOES IT TAKE?

You don't have to devote a big block of time to gentle exercise. Four 15-minute walks distributed throughout your day can be just as productive as a continuous hour of exercise. For most people, adding 30 to 60 minutes of gentle activity every day will do the job. Remember: *The more mitochondria you have, the more easily your body can burn body fat for fuel.* As it becomes easier to use up excess body fat, you'll lose weight more rapidly, move more easily, feel healthier, and become leaner.

Researchers at the University of Pittsburgh recently completed a study of 56 sedentary, overweight women. Each began walking and/or cycling five times a week for 40 minutes. Half of the women worked out continuously for 40 minutes; the other half divided their daily exercise into four 10-minute sessions.

After 20 weeks, both groups had boosted their aerobic capacity. But there was a significant difference. Not only did the women who exercised more often but for shorter periods adhere better to their exercise schedules, they also lost more weight.

It's important to create a schedule that works for you—one that allows time to do whatever exercise you plan for the day, whether in long or short sessions.

Why not take a 15-minute walk right now? Let yourself be pleased. Let yourself get moving. Feel the difference!

Lean for Life®
DAILY ACTION PLAN

PROTEIN DAY

Week ___I___   Day ___3___   Date _____

Time	Meal Plans	Serving Size	Carbs (grams)
_____	**Breakfast**		
	Protein		
	Beverage		
_____	**Protein Snack**		
_____	**Lunch**		
	Protein		
	Beverage		
_____	**Protein Snack**		
_____	**Dinner**		
	Protein		
	Beverage		
_____	**Protein Snack**		
		TOTAL	

Keto Reading _____
Weight _____
Vitamins   AM   Noon   PM
Water _____

Activities _____

Pedometer Steps _____

WEEKLY BODY MEASUREMENTS
Chest _____   Hips _____
Waist _____   Thighs _____
Abdomen _____

SUCCESS LEARNING TOOLS
Read pages # _____
Audio Tape _____
Video _____
CD-ROM _____
Bio-Card ™ _____
Affirmation _____

Other _____
Plan to Overcome Today's Obstacles:
_____
_____
_____
_____

Notes:
_____
_____
_____

**TODAY IS YOUR THIRD PROTEIN DAY
UNLESS OTHERWISE DIRECTED
BY YOUR HEALTH CARE PROFESSIONAL.**

STEP IT UP!

How much exercise did you do yesterday? What did you eat?

You can answer these questions because you're maintaining a Daily Action Plan. But most people have no clue as to how many calories they consume, how many steps they've taken, or how many additional calories they've burned through exercise and activity on a given day.

As reported in the *New England Journal of Medicine*, people consistently *underestimate* the number of calories they consume and *overestimate* the number of minutes they exercise. That's why it's important to have objective measurements of food intake and exercise.

Your Daily Action Plan is your tool for monitoring your food intake. A pedometer or step counter is an easy way to monitor your physical activity and daily exercise. You can purchase pedometers at most sporting goods or discount stores. Information on the Lean for Life pedometer/activity counter may be found in the Resources Section.

Once you have your pedometer, you'll clip it on your belt, waistband, or shoe every morning and record the number of steps you take on your Daily Action Plan before you go to bed.

Most Lindora patients aim for achieving 10,000 steps a day. If you've been only moderately active, it may take time to work up to that many steps. I've been wearing a pedometer nearly every day for three years. When I first started wearing it, I considered myself to be a fairly active person. I've always tried to take the stairs instead of elevators and I often walk around my office while I'm talking on the phone. My daughter, who was just one year old at the time, had just started walking, and keeping up with her seemed like a nonstop workout.

I was shocked to discover that I was only logging about 3,500 steps a day on my pedometer! I thought of myself as active, but I was almost a couch potato. That's when I made a conscious decision to become more active. I now check my pedometer several times a day. If the number is low and it looks like I won't make my goal of 8,000 to 10,000 steps for the day, I either take a 10-minute walk or stand at my desk and shift my weight from foot to foot for five or 10 minutes while I continue to work.

A pedometer not only measures steps, but it also reminds you to take those steps. After you wear a pedometer for a while, you, too, will come up with different ways to make sure you get the activity you need to become leaner and healthier.

Aim for success, not perfection. Make it your goal to gradually increase your number of steps—then see, feel, and record your progress.

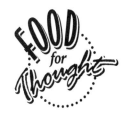

"The future belongs
to those who believe
in the beauty
of their dreams."

— Eleanor Roosevelt

WARMING UP: THE GENTLE EXERCISE SYSTEM

One especially effective way to begin enjoying the benefits of gentle exercise is to use *Warming Up: The Gentle Exercise System*. It's a fun, easy-to-use video program that you can do at your own pace and in the privacy, comfort, and convenience of your home. Our physicians prescribe *Warming Up* to help patients develop the habit of exercising at home in ways that are safe, enjoyable, and appropriate for their level of fitness.

The *Warming Up* video includes a 33-minute exercise class featuring "real people"—men and women of various ages and sizes. The booklet that accompanies the video helps users tailor the program to their individual needs. The program is especially appropriate for people who are overweight, obese, diabetic, arthritic, or who are suffering from a stress-related or chronic illness. *Warming Up* is also used successfully by serious athletes and other well-conditioned people who are returning to activity after childbirth, surgery, injury, or illness, or who want an enjoyable complement to their regular workouts or training sessions.

The remaining 20 minutes of the video provide an opportunity to meet the people in the exercise class and to hear the creator of the *Warming Up* system, Herman M. Frankel, M.D., speak directly to the viewer about the importance of establishing a gentle pace. A physician and teacher, Frankel has been internationally honored for his work with overweight and inactive people and is a holder of the U.S. Secretary of Human Services Award for Excellence, the nation's highest honor for community health promotion and disease prevention.

Regular users of the *Warming Up* system enjoy such benefits as:

❑ Increased ease and maintenance of weight loss

❑ Increased metabolic rate

❑ Increased ability to burn body fat for fuel

❑ Increased responsiveness to insulin

❑ Increased strength, flexibility, suppleness, and stability

❑ Increased balance, agility, and coordination

❑ Increased enjoyment of physical activity

❑ Relief from anxiety

❑ Control over depression

❑ Improved sleep

❑ Stimulation of circulation

❏ Normalization of appetite

❏ Lower blood pressure

❏ Improved lipid and carbohydrate metabolism

❏ Improved appearance

Warming Up has been extensively tested by physicians and other health professionals in a variety of clinical settings, including the Lindora Medical Clinics, where more than 10,000 of our patients have successfully used the video program as they learned to become Lean for Life. Information on ordering *Warming Up* is found in the Resources section of this book.

TODAY'S EATING PLAN

Q: What's my meal plan for today?

A: Are you in ketosis? If not, plan to make this your third Protein Day, and be sure to do your gentle exercise. If you are in ketosis, today can be your first "Menu Day". Go to the menu and choose your breakfast, lunch, and dinner. Be sure to have protein snacks available in case you feel hungry.

DAY 4

THOSE @#%&*! CRAVINGS

You can learn to deal effectively with the physical causes of cravings.

You're having a terrific day. You feel focused, positive, and in control. You've exercised and you're eating well. Then suddenly, without warning, it happens. A nagging temptation for one of your favorite foods grabs hold and refuses to let go. The more you try to ignore it, the more tormenting it becomes. You feel lightheaded, irritable, edgy. Your mouth waters. Minute by minute, your willpower erodes like a sandcastle at high tide.

Welcome to the world of cravings, where powerful forces stronger than mere willpower rule. Cravings can be your worst nightmare, undermining your self-esteem, shaking your self-confidence, and derailing your weight-loss program.

Cravings don't just happen. They're the result of various physical, psychological, and environmental factors that affect the way your body and brain function. Once you understand what causes them and how you can neutralize their impact, you'll have jumped a major hurdle on your journey to becoming Lean for Life.

One of the most common physical causes of cravings is an elevated "setpoint." If you just felt your eyes glazing over at the thought of reading "scientific stuff," stay with me. Cravings can be deadly to your weight-loss efforts, so anything you can learn—and do—to counter them will stack the deck in your favor.

YOUR SETPOINT AND HOW IT WORKS

The human body was designed to store fat and then burn it as fuel. Your body is an exquisitely designed machine, in which millions of cells function in perfect synchronicity. Your brain, digestive tract, muscles and fat all work together through a highly complex system of biochemical feedback loops to maintain a stable weight. In other words, these different parts of the body "talk" to each other, coordinating their efforts to maintain a stable weight. That particular weight, which your body strives to maintain, is commonly known as the "setpoint."

Think of your setpoint as a thermostat. Just as a thermostat works to maintain a constant temperature by regulating the heating or cooling system in response to outside conditions, the setpoint raises or lowers your appetite and metabolism—the rate at which your body burns calories—in response to how much you're eating.

This raises an obvious question. "If my body's designed to maintain a stable weight," you may be wondering, "why did I gain weight in the first place and why is it so #*@&%! hard to lose it?" Here's the deal. If you live in the desert and the temperature outside is 85 degrees, your home's cooling system will have no problem maintaining an indoor temperature of 72 degrees. But if it's a sweltering 120 degrees outside, the cooling system will eventually become overtaxed. It won't be able to function adequately, so it will start maintaining the indoor temperature at higher than 72 degrees.

In essence, the same is true with your body. If you eat more calories and/or get too little exercise over a long enough period of time, your body's

CATHY   **By Cathy Guisewite**

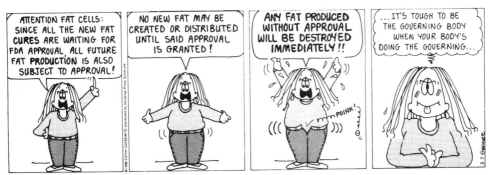

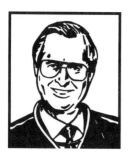

DR. STAMPER

"There are many
benefits to remaining
in ketosis. One of
the greatest is a
dramatic reduction in
hunger. You'll
eat less because you'll
want less."

weight regulation system won't be able to cope adequately. It will adjust upward and your body's systems will "settle in" to support a higher weight.

So what happens when you start to lose weight? Because your body strives for equilibrium, its metabolic alarm system goes off as soon as you stop eating as much as you normally do. Your body demands food. Like the ravenous, man-eating plant in *Little Shop of Horrors*, it has one thing on it's mind: "Feed me! Feed me!" You begin feeling uncomfortable, anxious, perhaps even edgy. The quickest form of relief? That's right—food! And thus, the cycle of losing and regaining continues.

Dr. Stamper has told patients for years that dieters don't fail because of a lack of willpower—they fail because of cravings. As long as your setpoint remains elevated, you will crave food whenever your body senses you're not eating enough to maintain your present weight.

As you can imagine, these mental "hunger alarms" make it especially difficult for overweight people to lose weight—and even tougher for them to keep it off. Your body will fight to hold on to whatever excess fat it has become accustomed to. It will also do its best to replace any weight you happen to lose. That's why it's essential to understand the nature of your food cravings and how to control them.

SO WHAT'S THE SOLUTION?

Here are three powerful short-term tools for immediate relief from cravings, as well as a fourth that yields both short-term and long-term benefits:

1. Since you'll be limiting your carbohydrates during the weight-loss phase of the program, your body will be using your stored fat as its primary fuel source. Throughout the program we'll refer to the physiological state of burning fat as "ketosis." Two of the benefits of being in ketosis are a dramatic reduction in hunger and fewer cravings.

2. Medications are now available for short-term use to help control food cravings that may result from fluctuating serotonin levels. Serotonin is a powerful neurotransmitter that regulates mood, hunger, and eating behavior. When serotonin levels are elevated in your hypothalamus— the appetite control center of the brain— you may feel less hungry and experience fewer cravings. Consult your physician as to whether such medications may help you.

3. Stress management tools, such as mental training exercises, a 15-minute walk and the neck massage technique you'll learn later next week all help provide immediate relief from cravings by naturally modifying your biochemistry.

4. The gentle exercise strategies we discussed yesterday benefit your muscle cells in two important ways. First, you develop more mitochrondria in your muscles through gentle exercise, which increases your ability to burn fat. You also develop more insulin receptors on the surface of the cells, which improves your body's ability to move sugar from the bloodstream into your muscle cells. This helps to stabilize blood sugar levels, which in turn lessens cravings.

Tomorrow, we'll explore another cause of cravings to see how people, places, and events can stimulate your food cravings—and what you can do to stay focused and in control.

TODAY'S EATING PLAN

Today and for the remainder of Week One, you'll be following the "Menu Plan." (See pages 31 through 34.)

Another Lean for Life Success Story

"My food cravings used to be relentless. I've made more midnight runs to the market than I care to admit. One night I was in line at a convenience store behind a guy who was buying a pint of vodka. His hands were trembling, and I remember feeling pity for him. Then it dawned on me that we really weren't that different. After all, I had gotten out of bed in the middle of the night to buy a pint of my own— double fudge brownie ice cream. Now that I've done the Lean for Life program, I experience cravings a lot less often. And when I do, I know what to do about it."

—Jody

KETOSIS + EXERCISE = INCREASED WEIGHT LOSS

The more you're in ketosis and the more steps you take, the more weight you can expect to lose.

That's the finding of a 1995 research project conducted by Jan Hunter, R.N., Lindora's Director of Nursing Services and Clinic Operations; Jayme Davidson, R.N.; Deena Eshom, L.V.N.; Vickie Flatt, L.V.N.; and Carolyn Lehm, R.N.

The six-month study of 6,032 Lindora patients found that:

...those who were in ketosis more than 90% of the time—and recorded more than 25,000 steps per week—averaged a 3.2 pound weekly weight loss, while participants who were in ketosis less than 60% of the time—and logged less than 25,000 steps per week—averaged a 1.9 pound weekly weight loss.

The bottom line? Participants who were in ketosis more than 90% of the time—and averaged 25,000 or more steps per week—*lost 60% more weight* than those who logged fewer than 25,000 and were in ketosis less than 60% of the time. To maximize your weight loss results, stay in ketosis and keep moving!

WHY WALK?

When you walk, you:

- ❑ Improve your fat-burning capacity
- ❑ Improve your carbohydrate metabolism (increased insulin receptors)
- ❑ Improve your cardiovascular fitness (enhance circulation, heart and lung function, delivery of blood and oxygen to cells)
- ❑ Improve your mood (endorphins, your body's "feel-good" chemical, are released)
- ❑ Improve stress resilience (your ability to offset effects of stress hormones)
- ❑ Improve your ability to enjoy solitude
- ❑ Provide time for yourself to reflect, ponder and think

Lean for Life®
DAILY ACTION PLAN

Week _____ Day _____ Date _____

Time	Meal Plans	Serving Size	Carbs (grams)
	Breakfast		
	Protein		
	Fruit or grain		
	Beverage		
	Protein Snack		
	Lunch		
	Protein		
	Vegetable		
	Lettuce		
	Fruit		
	Beverage		
	Miscellaneous		
	Protein Snack		
	Dinner		
	Protein		
	Vegetable		
	Lettuce		
	Fruit		
	Beverage		
	Miscellaneous		
	Protein Snack		
		TOTAL	

Keto Reading _____
Weight _____
Vitamins   AM _____ Noon _____ PM _____
Water _____

Activities _____
_____
_____

Pedometer Steps _____

WEEKLY BODY MEASUREMENTS
Chest _____   Hips _____
Waist _____   Thighs _____
Abdomen _____

SUCCESS LEARNING TOOLS
Read pages # _____
Audio Tape _____
Video _____
CD-ROM _____
Bio-Card ™ _____
Affirmation _____

Other _____
Plan to Overcome Today's Obstacles:
_____
_____
_____
_____
_____

Notes:
_____
_____
_____
_____

CHOOSE ONE DAY EACH WEEK AS YOUR "PROTEIN DAY."

STOP!

Whenever you're tempted to do anything that might interfere with your program, *STOP*:

STOP! Visualize a stop sign and hear the word "stop." Immediately stop what you're doing!

TAKE a deep, cleansing breath. This creates a "window of opportunity" during which you can become aware of the temptation you're facing and can start over.

OBSERVE your situation, yourself, and your options. What's going on? How are you feeling? Are you hungry, angry, lonely, tired? What are you wanting? What are you needing? What really matters to you? What choices do you have? What actions will help you move toward what's really important to you?

PLAN of Action. Choose a Plan of Action based on one or more of the options available to you and put that plan into operation. Shift the focus away from food by doing something: taking a walk, calling a friend, sitting quietly for five minutes and letting your attention rest on your breathing, going window shopping, listening to music, working on a project, or reviewing your Motivator cards to remind yourself why becoming Lean for Life is important to you.

If you find yourself thinking "I'm tired of not eating what I want—I'm going to have a treat!" make an active choice to focus on the benefits of maintaining your Plan of Action. Let yourself hear whatever voices inside of you are suggesting that you abandon or sabotage your Lean for Life program, and pause long enough to acknowledge and respond to those voices. Encourage yourself as you would a close friend.

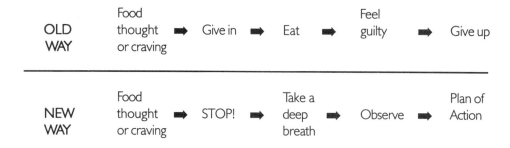

OLD WAY	Food thought or craving	➡	Give in	➡	Eat	➡	Feel guilty	➡	Give up
NEW WAY	Food thought or craving	➡	STOP!	➡	Take a deep breath	➡	Observe	➡	Plan of Action

The more often you do this, the more easily and effectively you'll be able to do it. That's because after you do something successfully again and again, it starts becoming spontaneous and natural. It becomes part of you. It becomes a habit.

ANY QUESTIONS?

Q: Can I use one of the protein snacks or products instead of a meal?

A: It's fine to use protein snacks occasionally in place of lean meats, fish, and other choices from your protein list. When you do, count it as your protein serving. For long-term success, however, it's important for you to learn how to plan, shop for, and prepare appropriate meals.

Q: Do I really need to take the vitamins so often?

A: Yes! The vitamin and mineral supplements help ensure that your body is getting the nutrients it needs—and that you'll continue feeling and looking healthy!

Q: Can I substitute certain foods on the menu with foods that have the same number of calories?

A: No. You need to follow the nutritional menu carefully to ensure that you're receiving proper nutrition while achieving maximum weight loss. Foods that may have the same number of calories may be higher in carbohydrates than those featured in the program.

Q: Refresh my memory! What are the major benefits of staying in ketosis?

A: When you're in mild to moderate ketosis, you'll lose weight rapidly and safely. You'll feel less hungry, less often. Your cravings will diminish. You'll have more energy and a greater sense of well-being. Most important, you'll burn excess body fat as rapidly as possible, while maintaining lean muscle mass.

DAY 5

CRAVINGS CAUSED BY PEOPLE, PLACES, EMOTIONS AND EVENTS

You can learn to change the way you respond to the forces and factors that trigger cravings.

How many times have you gone to the movies and suddenly found yourself craving popcorn? Even if you weren't hungry, your past experiences, the unmistakable aroma, the sound of kernels popping, and the sight of others eating were enough to lure you toward the concession stand.

Some people call this "Pavlovian conditioning." Back in the late 19th century, Russian scientist Ivan Pavlov conducted an experiment in which he sounded a bell when giving food to his dogs. After repeating the experiment many times, Pavlov's four-legged friends began to associate eating with the sound of the bell. They would salivate every time the bell rang, even when no food was present.

Like it or not, we have more in common with Pavlov's dogs than we might like to admit. We, too, have been conditioned, both personally and by society, to respond to certain emotions, events, and people by eating.

When you have a "conditioned response," you react without thinking. While certain conditioned responses tend to be universal—eating and drinking to excess during holidays and celebrations, for example—each of us also has unique conditioned responses. If you had a grandmother who made caramel apples every Halloween, it's a safe bet you'll develop a desire for them in late October. If your mother made hot cranberry cider every time you had a ticklish throat, odds are you're going to develop a sudden appetite for that brew the next time you're feeling sick.

CHANGING HOW YOU RESPOND

It's often difficult to permanently remove or change these cues, but you can learn how to change the ways you respond to them.

The following strategies will help you:

1. *Observe your behavior.* Identifying your conditioned responses is the first step in reprogramming them. When you're at the movies, for example, and you just "have to have popcorn," recognize what's happening. Eating popcorn at the movies is a reaction, a habit, but you don't *have* to have it. When you shift your focus away from self-defeating behavior, you'll be taking a huge step toward remaining in control. Focus instead on the film you're watching and the people you're with.

2. *Get active.* Whatever you do, don't sit and brood about how intense your cravings are. There's great truth in the adage "action equals power." Shift your attention to activities other than eating. Take a walk. Go for a swim. Head for the gym. Call a friend spur-of-the-moment and go dancing. At Lindora, we call these kinds of activities "Biomodifiers™," because they can actually change your brain and body chemistry. We'll talk more about Biomodifiers on Day 9.

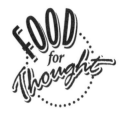

"If we all did the things we are capable of doing, we would literally astonish ourselves."

—Thomas Edison

DRABBLE   By Kevin Fagan

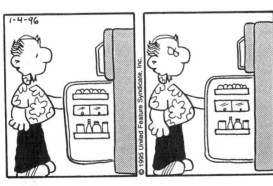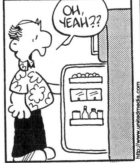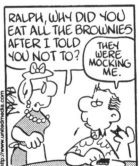

DRABBLE reprinted by permission of United Feature Syndicate, Inc.

3. *Consider the consequences*. Think ahead to tomorrow. Ask yourself how you'll feel physically and mentally if you give in to your cravings today. Do you really want to "wear" that piece of chocolate cake? Are you willing to exercise more to burn all those extra calories?

4. *Delay your gratification*. Cravings are like gnats. Some of them will pester you for what seems like forever, but most of them can be shooed away. The next time you're overcome with a craving, make a deal with yourself. Delay your reaction for a given period of time—an hour, three hours, one day. Tell yourself that if the craving is still as strong, you'll deal with it then. More often than not, cravings diminish or even pass within an hour or two. This is one of those rare occasions when stall tactics can be productive.

5. *Consider alternatives*. A craving is a suggestion, not a command. Just because the notion of stuffing yourself with cherry pie crosses your mind doesn't mean you have to actually *do* it. Whenever you feel like acting impulsively, pause long enough to explore what you're really feeling and thinking. You're likely to discover alternatives that are far more nourishing.

CONTROLLING CRAVINGS: HOW TO RESPOND TO ENVIRONMENTAL CUES

Here are several steps you can take to deal more effectively with those times that spark your desire to eat:

❑ *Control the number of times you eat every day*. If a snack helps curb your appetite, build one into your Daily Action Plan. If you can structure your eating, you'll find yourself eating less and enjoying it more.

❑ *Be sure to eat breakfast*. Many overweight people skip breakfast and justify it as "saving calories." Those who achieve and maintain long-term weight loss almost always eat a healthy breakfast and find doing so makes it easier to control their appetite later in the day.

❑ *Choose one or two places in your house where you will eat*. When you snack, go to one of your eating places and eat it. If you get the urge to nibble while watching TV, wait until your program is over, then have your meal in one of your special places.

Lean *for* Life®
DAILY ACTION PLAN

Week _____ **Day** _____ **Date** _____

Time	Meal Plans	Serving Size	Carbs (grams)
	Breakfast		
	Protein		
	Fruit or grain		
	Beverage		
	Protein Snack		
	Lunch		
	Protein		
	Vegetable		
	Lettuce		
	Fruit		
	Beverage		
	Miscellaneous		
	Protein Snack		
	Dinner		
	Protein		
	Vegetable		
	Lettuce		
	Fruit		
	Beverage		
	Miscellaneous		
	Protein Snack		
		TOTAL	

Keto Reading _____

Weight _____

Vitamins   AM _____ Noon _____ PM _____

Water _____

Activities _____
_____
_____

Pedometer Steps _____

WEEKLY BODY MEASUREMENTS

Chest _____ Hips _____

Waist _____ Thighs _____

Abdomen _____

SUCCESS LEARNING TOOLS

Read pages # _____

Audio Tape _____

Video _____

CD-ROM _____

Bio-Card™ _____

Affirmation _____

_____

Other _____

Plan to Overcome Today's Obstacles:
_____
_____
_____
_____
_____

Notes: _____
_____
_____
_____

CHOOSE ONE DAY EACH WEEK AS YOUR "PROTEIN DAY."

6. *Review your reasons for becoming lean*. Remind yourself why you made a commitment to becoming Lean for Life. Continue reviewing the Motivator cards you prepared on Day 1. They're an effective tool to help maintain your enthusiasm and deal effectively with the people, places, emotions, and events that trigger your response to eat.

7. *If it's really an urge to chew, then do*. The next time you experience a craving, ask yourself whether you're craving food or if what you really want is simply to chew. Often, one has little to do with the other.

    If you're feeling tense and angry, for example, you may find yourself craving crunchy foods. This "mouth hunger" can be satisfied without jeopardizing your program. Many of the Lean for Life snacks have a firm, chewy consistency. Cut one into small pieces and eat it slowly, over a 20-minute period, drinking water between bites. This will satisfy your hunger as well as your desire to chew. Also try sugarless gum. You can chew as much as you want without blowing your diet!

The cues for cravings are all around us. How you respond to them is up to you. You're a person with goals and insight. You—not the TV, not the pastry shop, not other people—can decide what, when, and how much you'll eat.

Another Lean for Life Success Story

"I know I'm really stressed whenever I crave sweets. I get that gnawing feeling that sends me searching. I remember one time I was rifling through purses I hadn't used for months, hoping to find a piece of candy. Now that I understand what's going on, I take a deep breath and ask myself, 'What is it that I really want? Will eating really make me feel better?' The urgency usually passes, and I'm fine. These days, when I have a piece of candy, it's because I've made a conscious choice to do so."

— Cynthia

THEN&NOW

Your Turn

Which people, places and events trigger *your* desire to eat? What foods do you find yourself craving in various situations? Examples: "When I'm busy, I crave greasy fast food, so instead I could have an 'emergency supply' of protein bars with me..." "When I'm at a ballgame, I crave hot dogs and beer, so instead I could take some turkey jerky with me..."

When I:	I crave:	Instead, I could:
_____	_____	_____
_____	_____	_____
_____	_____	_____
_____	_____	_____
_____	_____	_____

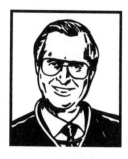

DR. STAMPER

"Your Daily Action Plan will show you how many carbohydrates you can tolerate each day without interrupting your ketosis and your continued weight loss."

ANY QUESTIONS?

Q: *What you call environmental cues have been my downfall for years. Now that I'm aware of them, I feel much more in control. Do you have any tips for maintaining that control?*

A: These success strategies will help conquer cravings caused by environmental cues:

❑   One of the best ways to break the connection between the sight of your favorite food (an external cue) and your automatic desire to eat is not to have the food around in the first place. Eliminate as many temptations as possible. Do an inventory of your kitchen. If you find foods you don't want to be eating while you're on the program, consider giving them away or throwing them out.

❑   Remove the candy jar from the coffee table. Retire the cookie jar to a storage unit or the top shelf above the refrigerator. If they're not "staring at you," you'll be less likely to react to them out of habit. Out of sight, out of mind, out of mouth!

❑   Avoid your "danger zones." You can bolster your self-control by avoiding places you know will prompt you to eat. If the candy machine in the office break room is your downfall, take your break outdoors. If your favorite fast-food restaurant lies in wait for you on your drive home, avoid the ambush by taking an alternate route.

❑   Become independent and creative. Whenever you feel tempted, remember that one of the benefits of greater awareness is greater independence. Use these occasions as reminders that you're now *acting mindfully* rather than *reacting mindlessly*.

THE DENIAL TRAP

You'll understand what a powerful force denial can be—and how to overcome it.

I t wasn't too many years ago that my friend Mary Beth called from her car phone to let me know she was running a few minutes late for our lunch meeting. She had stopped by her favorite department store to try on a dress and was totally exasperated.

"I swear those people must be having their clothes made in Munchkinland!" she later declared as she dragged an onion ring through the mayonnaise that had dripped from her cheeseburger. "They're cutting their clothes smaller all the time. Their size 10 used to fit me like a glove. Now I can barely fit into a 14!"

Today, Mary Beth looks back on that conversation and laughs. She now jokes that she was a real "denial diva." It's a description that, unlike the dress, fit her perfectly.

Denial is an unwillingness or refusal to accept or admit life's realities. The difference between lying and denial is simple. Lying is actively hiding the truth from others. Denial is actively hiding the truth from ourselves.

WHY DENY?

Denial protects us from a truth that may be painful. After all, as long as we're in denial, there's no problem. And if there's no problem, then there's no need to seek solutions. Until you understand what a powerful force denial can be, you're likely to find yourself doomed to play the no-win diet game, taking two steps forward and two steps back.

Most of us have developed a variety of ways to protect ourselves from the truth. So when we decide to make significant changes in the way we think and act, it's important that we also become aware of the hidden mental patterns that block our progress and keep us mired in those unproductive patterns and behaviors.

Because we're often unaware that such patterns exist, it can be a real challenge to overcome them. At Lindora, we refer to denial and other self-protective behaviors as "defensive barriers." Another defensive barrier that often gets in the way of lasting weight loss is rationalization, which we'll take a look at tomorrow.

Recognizing and disarming defensive barriers such as denial isn't easy. In fact, it's one of those classic "Catch-22" challenges: In order to address a problem, you first have to acknowledge that there *is* a problem. Yet if you're deep in denial, it's unlikely you're going to recognize or acknowledge that you are.

BREAKING THE "INSANITY CYCLE"

Do *you* ever do the same thing over and over again and expect a different result?

While even rats in a maze eventually figure out which paths are the express lanes to nowhere, people aren't always quite so quick to get the picture. That's why the Lean for Life program focuses on changing the way you *think* as much as the way you *eat*.

To make lasting changes, first you need to gain a new awareness of how you think and how that thought process may be leading you directly down a dead-end path. Once you identify and begin eliminating your defensive barriers—those subtle, subconscious self-sabotage strategies that help keep you stuck—you'll be one step closer to shedding those pounds and *keeping* them off for life.

Lean for Life®
DAILY ACTION PLAN

Week _____   Day _____   Date _____

Keto Reading _____
Weight _____
Vitamins   AM   Noon   PM
Water _____

Activities _____
_____
_____
_____

Pedometer Steps

WEEKLY BODY MEASUREMENTS

Chest _____   Hips _____
Waist _____   Thighs _____
Abdomen _____

SUCCESS LEARNING TOOLS

Read pages # _____
Audio Tape _____
Video _____
CD-ROM _____
Bio-Card™ _____
Affirmation _____
_____

Other _____
Plan to Overcome Today's Obstacles:
_____
_____
_____
_____

Notes: _____
_____
_____
_____

CHOOSE ONE DAY EACH WEEK AS YOUR "PROTEIN DAY."

Time	Meal Plans	Serving Size	Carbs (grams)
	Breakfast		
	Protein		
	Fruit or grain		
	Beverage		
	Protein Snack		
	Lunch		
	Protein		
	Vegetable		
	Lettuce		
	Fruit		
	Beverage		
	Miscellaneous		
	Protein Snack		
	Dinner		
	Protein		
	Vegetable		
	Lettuce		
	Fruit		
	Beverage		
	Miscellaneous		
	Protein Snack		
		TOTAL	

DISARMING DENIAL

Many people are convinced they don't have any real power over their lives. What they don't realize is that by making conscious changes in the way they *think*, they can change the way they *live*.

Making a conscious decision to break the cycle is the first step toward achieving your goal. If you want different results, you must start doing things differently. The first step is becoming more fully aware of your power to recognize and dismantle your defensive barriers and change the way you think. Until you do, your power is nothing more than unrealized potential.

In his book *The Unfair Advantage*, psychologist Tom Miller shares an analogy of a horse and rider that beautifully illustrates the relationship that exists between the conscious and the subconscious mind.

Horses are magnificent creatures. Their intelligence, however, is limited. Once a horse becomes accustomed to turning west at the first fork in the trail, convincing it to head east can become a true battle of will. The horse, being a creature of habit, will come to a stubborn standstill right in the middle of the road rather than change its routine.

But with the right strategy and plenty of patience and determination, a skilled rider can change the horse's habits, retraining it to move with grace in whatever direction the rider chooses. Even though the horse is physically bigger, the rider is mentally stronger.

WALKING: IT BENEFITS YOUR BODY *AND* YOUR BRAIN

Did you know that taking a brisk walk can actually help you think faster? Studies by Robert Dustman, director of the Neuropsychology Research Laboratory at the Veterans Affairs Medical Center Center in Salt Lake City, Utah, show that while active, aerobically fit adults over 60 retain much of the quick-wittedness of youth, adults over 40 who *don't* exercise develop undernourished neurons in their brains and don't move electrical signals as quickly. As a result, their minds slow down!

This sneak peak at "BioModifiers"—experiences or activities that can change your brain chemistry—is just one example of how you can use the mind-body connection to your advantage. We'll talk more about "BioMod" on Day 9.

Your Turn

As you read today's feature, you may have found yourself thinking "I never do that!" Take the following quiz. Every "Yes" answer would suggest that perhaps sometimes you *do*.

1. Do you ever refuse to weigh yourself because you'd rather not know? (The "What I Don't Know Won't Hurt Me" approach doesn't help avoid pain; it only delays it.)

2. Have you ever blamed the clothes dryer for tighter-fitting clothes? (Unless everyone else in your family has the same problem, this should tell you something.)

3. Do you avoid mirrors, especially when getting out of the shower?

4. Do you ever eat junk food while alone (at home or in the car) and make a point to throw away the candy, cookie, and potato chip wrappers before anyone else sees them?

5. Have you ever blamed your weight problem on "thyroid trouble," "big bones," or a "slow metabolism," even though you've never had a medical examination that supports your theories?

6. Do you ever exaggerate how long, how often, or how hard you exercise?

7. Do you blame bloat and excess weight on "water retention" resulting from your period, getting ready to begin your period, or having just had your period? (This is an especially questionable excuse if you are male!)

WHO'S IN CHARGE HERE?

Like the rider, *you*—the aware, awake, mindful you—want to be in charge of your journey. You want to be the one who decides where you're going, which route you'll travel, and how long it will take to get there. You want to have the courage to examine your motives, understand your reactions, and learn life lessons along the way.

The Lean for Life program is about gaining mastery over yourself so that you're in control. The affirmations and other mental training techniques you'll encounter in this book are effective ways to gain that mastery. At Lindora, we call this process "thought control."

Some people react strongly to this concept. The words evoke images of manipulation, as in "I don't want anyone but me controlling my thoughts!"

That's exactly the point. True thought control is not about surrendering power to anyone. It's about claiming it for yourself. By becoming more self-aware and by consciously using the mental training strategies featured in this program, you can learn to reframe your thoughts so that they are more helpful to you. When you do this consistently, new habits will emerge. You'll have an opportunity to explore thought control more in depth on Day 10.

This program has been designed for lifelong success. If you find yourself thinking that some of the procedures or information don't apply to you (we call this the "Not Me" Syndrome) or if you begin to discount or ignore vital

Another Lean for Life Success Story

THEN&NOW

"Defensive barriers are like blinders. You don't see the big picture. When my defensive barriers are up, immediate gratification is all that matters. I want it and I want it now. They lull you into believing that whatever you eat today doesn't matter as long as you promise to buckle down tomorrow. But until you finally break that cycle, tomorrow never comes."

—*Marcia*

WHAT THELMA LEARNED

Thelma was discouraged and confused.

She had been on the program for more than a week, yet she hadn't lost a pound and wasn't in ketosis.

"Maybe my body is just different," Thelma speculated. "I don't know what to say."

When Jill, one of our clinic nurses, offered to review Thelma's Daily Action Plans with her, Thelma said she wasn't "a detail person" and didn't "have time" to write down what she ate and drank every day.

While telling Jill that she had been "doing the program to the letter," Thelma poured herself a cup of coffee and added three spoons of non-dairy creamer.

She must have noticed Jill's expression.

"Oh, don't worry," Thelma said. "This is the 'lite' stuff."

It didn't take Sherlock Holmes to solve this mystery. Jill pointed out that while the "lite" non-dairy creamer had less fat, it contained the same number of calories and double the carbohydrates! Thelma was consuming 150 extra calories and 30 extra grams of carbohydrate every day without realizing it!

The bottom line? Eliminate any mystery by writing down everything you eat and drink, every day, throughout "Phase 1: Weight Loss." Your Daily Action Plan is a valuable resource that allows you to identify any errors and correct them immediately.

---

features of the program, it's a clear warning sign that your defensive barriers—rationalizations and denial—are firmly in place.

Don't be surprised if you find yourself resisting change along the way. In fact, expect it. People often have a definite resistance to doing things that are different from what they've done before, even when they realize that what they've done in the past no longer works. In the coming weeks, you'll discover that it's possible to overcome the mental barriers and find a new, more rewarding path.

ANY QUESTIONS?

Q: *Can I save a fruit serving from one meal and eat it later?*

A: Since one of the goals of the program is to help you learn to eat nutritious, high-fiber foods at regular intervals, it's important that you eat all the designated foods at the designated times.

Q: *Why is bread limited to whole grain with 70 calories or fewer per slice?*

A: Other kinds of bread are too high in calories and/or too low in fiber and certain nutrients.

Q: *Why are some meats and fish not on the menu?*

A: They're too high in natural fat and calories.

"MR. MITO" SAYS:

"People often ask, "How often—and how long—should I walk?" Our own research shows that for inactive people, almost any addition of steps to their existing routine enhances mood, energy level, sleep, and weight loss.

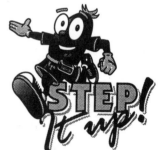

Three 10-minute walks a day is a realistic initial goal for almost everyone. Since walking is one of those human activities in which more is better, aim to increase your duration and distance a little every day or every other day."

RECOGNIZING RATIONALIZATION

*You'll discover the benefits of changing
the way you think as well as
the way you eat.*

When Steve returned home from work early one afternoon to find Paula eating fast-food fried chicken, he finally understood why his wife had been struggling on her weight-loss program.

As always, Paula attempted to joke her way out of the situation. When it came to creative excuses, she was in a league of her own.

"It's not what you think," she insisted as she licked her fingers. "I'm just moisturizing my skin from the inside out."

When Steve didn't even smirk, Paula got testy.

"Lighten up!" she said. "It was just two tiny pieces. And anyway, I don't look that bad for a 46-year-old woman with four kids!"

Paula's ability to rationalize is hardly unique. Our defensive barriers come to the rescue whenever we want or need to protect ourselves from unpleasant feelings, difficult situations, and painful truths. Like the quills of a porcupine, these barriers are not always raised, but they're always ready if needed. They have their purpose and they serve it well.

No one would dispute that our brains are wired to protect us from physical threats. When you're at a baseball game and a foul ball zooms in your direction, you don't *think* about how to react. You duck. When you

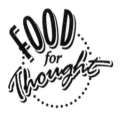

hear a loud, sudden sound, you flinch. Your eyes snap shut at an explosion of bright light. These reactions are instinctive and involuntary.

But the subtle ways in which we protect ourselves from emotional threats are much less obvious. We often react defensively, as Paula did, whenever we sense an attack on our self-image or on our worth and value as a person. Like a flinch or a blink of the eye, these reactions aren't the result of any conscious decision. In fact, we're usually not even aware of what we're doing.

One of the most common defensive barriers is rationalization. Rationalizations are excuses our minds make to help us feel better about a situation. When we rationalize, we justify our actions without acknowledging our responsibility for what has happened.

Because rationalizations are usually plausible, we can easily fool ourselves into believing them. This dilemma presents one of the greatest challenges of behavior change: How can we break a pattern when we're not even conscious it exists?

For starters, awareness is essential. Since our defensive barriers undermine our ability to change old habits, recognizing them is a fundamental step toward lasting success. To neutralize the negative impact that denial and rationalization can have in your life, use the following success strategies:

1. *Accept that your defensive barriers exist*. It's impossible to do any weight-loss program successfully without coming face-to-face with your defensive barriers. If they go unrecognized, they will prevent you from achieving your goals, and you may never know why you failed.

2. *Understand the damage defensive barriers have created for you and replace them with healthier patterns*. Look at your past weight-

CATHY

By Cathy Guisewite

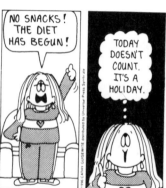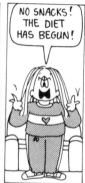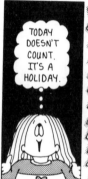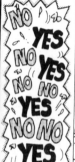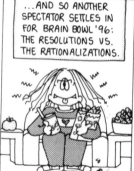

loss experiences to become more aware of how you've used rationalizations and denial to justify overeating. Can you think of one example of each? What influence did they have on your behavior? Did they really protect you or did they harm you? Knowing what you now know, what could you have done to neutralize their power?

3. *Exercise thought control.* At Lindora, we define thought control as the process in which you consciously recognize a negative or unproductive thought and immediately replace it with a positive, productive one. If you're thinking, "I want a hot fudge sundae!" substitute that thought with a conscious statement such as "I want to be lean, and every day when I make conscious choices, I'm getting closer to my goal." The process of thought control reminds you that your actions have consequences.

   By exercising thought control often enough, you can change your thoughts and feelings into patterns that will help rather than hinder you. Remember that inner voice we talked about on Day 2? As you become more skilled at thought control, it will become your cheerleader. Rather than urging you to have "just one piece," it can be trained to raise the red flag and ask "What are you doing?" Carefully consider what you really want before making a decision. Ask yourself: "Is eating this now going to get me what I want and need?"

4. *Understand that disarming defensive barriers is a process.* Even after you fully understand how rationalizations and denial get in your way, there are still going to be times when your resistance may be down and they'll get the best of you. When this happens, acknowledge that you've slipped, learn what you can from the experience, and accept that you made a choice that you wouldn't necessarily make again. Sometimes, the lessons we learn from our mistakes are well worth the price we pay.

5. *Remember that there may be a part of you that still resists change.* The familiar is comforting even when it is self-defeating. It can be challenging to do things differently, even when we realize what we've done in the past doesn't work.

6. *Be conscious of the "Not Me" Syndrome.* As you proceed with your program, pay careful attention to your thoughts and actions. Instead of saying "I never do that!" and discounting the advice, try following it. You may find that your defensive barriers have been keeping you away from the truth.

SOUND FAMILIAR?

To appreciate how often rationalizations creep into our everyday lives, review the following and check off any of those you can remember using:

- ❏ "I deserve this. I've been good all day!"
- ❏ "Oh, it's just a little bite."
- ❏ "There are starving children in (fill in name of country)."
- ❏ "It's a shame to waste food."
- ❏ "It's Friday night."
- ❏ "It's Saturday."
- ❏ "It's Sunday."
- ❏ "It's my birthday."
- ❏ "It's fat-free."
- ❏ "I'm on vacation."
- ❏ "I paid for it, I'm eating it."
- ❏ "I'm not feeling well. I've got to eat."
- ❏ "This diet isn't good for me."
- ❏ "If I don't eat I'm going to waste away to nothing!"
- ❏ "I don't know how to make healthy foods."
- ❏ "My friend eats this and doesn't gain weight."
- ❏ "I look pretty good for my age."
- ❏ "It's a holiday."
- ❏ "It would be rude not to eat it after she made it especially for me."
- ❏ "It's no big deal."
- ❏ "I didn't eat breakfast."
- ❏ "I'll make up for it tomorrow at the gym."

How good does a rationalization have to be to work? Only good enough to lull you into temptation or to let you off the hook. Any excuse is good enough when you're looking for a reason to eat.

Lean *for* Life®
DAILY ACTION PLAN

Week _____   Day _____   Date _____

Time	Meal Plans	Serving Size	Carbs (grams)
	Breakfast		
	Protein		
	Fruit or grain		
	Beverage		
	Protein Snack		
	Lunch		
	Protein		
	Vegetable		
	Lettuce		
	Fruit		
	Beverage		
	Miscellaneous		
	Protein Snack		
	Dinner		
	Protein		
	Vegetable		
	Lettuce		
	Fruit		
	Beverage		
	Miscellaneous		
	Protein Snack		
		TOTAL	

Keto Reading _____
Weight _____
Vitamins   AM   Noon   PM
Water _____

Activities _____
_____
_____

Pedometer Steps _____

WEEKLY BODY MEASUREMENTS
Chest _____   Hips _____
Waist _____   Thighs _____
Abdomen _____

SUCCESS LEARNING TOOLS
Read pages # _____
Audio Tape _____
Video _____
CD-ROM _____
Bio-Card ™ _____
Affirmation _____

Other _____
Plan to Overcome Today's Obstacles: _____
_____
_____
_____
_____
_____

Notes: _____
_____
_____
_____

CHOOSE ONE DAY EACH WEEK AS YOUR "PROTEIN DAY."

HOW ARE YOU DOING?

So how do you feel about your experience on the program after the first week?

Take some time to review the past week's Daily Action Plans. Are there any changes you want to incorporate in your program as you move into Week 2? More activity? Fewer snacks? More fluids? Less rationalization?

Jot down the changes and improvements you can make to enhance your results in the coming weeks.

_____

_____

_____

_____

_____

_____

_____

_____

The fine tuning you do now can have an impact on your results later!

YOUR WEEKLY PROTEIN DAY

Beginning with your second week of Weight Loss and continuing throughout your Lean for Life program, you'll choose one day each week as your Protein Day. Many people choose Monday, as it helps them get their week off to a great start and keeps them focused on their goal.

"WHAT IF MY KETOSTICK IS NEGATIVE?"

You'll be checking your ketostick for color every day during "Phase 1: Weight Loss." If your stick doesn't show pink to purple color, immediately do one to three Protein Days. This will help you get back into ketosis as quickly as possible. As soon as you're in ketosis again, resume the "Phase 1: Weight Loss" nutritional menu.

4

WEIGHT LOSS
WEEK TWO

THE MORE ENTHUSED, THE MORE YOU LOSE

You'll learn how your level of interest and enthusiasm directly impacts your degree of success.

Setting a goal is the easy part. Just ask anyone who's ever made a New Year's resolution. You begin with determination and a dream—to pay off your credit cards, to write the great American novel, to travel, to lose weight. You know what you want and vow that this time, you'll make it happen. And for a while, you do what it takes.

But then something happens. Your enthusiasm ebbs. Your focus becomes fuzzy and your determination dims. You don't give up, but you find yourself giving in. Excuses that would have never worked a week earlier are suddenly good enough. Today becomes tomorrow, and before you know it, you're back where you started, only more discouraged than before.

Sound familiar? We've all been there. Change is never easy. Consistent effort over an extended period of time isn't easy, either. If it were, we could erase the word "challenge" from the dictionary. But change *is* possible. Just ask any of the people whose inspiring success stories are included in this book. Every one of them knows an important secret: your level of interest and enthusiasm directly impacts your success. In other words, the more enthused, the more

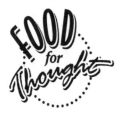

you'll lose. The more motivated you are, the more likely you will be to achieve your goal.

The challenge, of course, is maintaining your motivation over the long haul. To fully appreciate just how true this is, ask yourself the following questions:

❑ What was my goal on my last diet?

❑ Did I achieve the goal? How close did I come?

❑ How long did my enthusiasm last before I began making excuses and altering my program?

❑ How long did I maintain the weight loss I achieved?

On this program—as in life—your continued level of motivation is an important contributor to your success. It's rarely the most talented or even the luckiest person who succeeds. More often than not, those who win in life are those who stay committed and focused on the goal while others get sidetracked. Winners understand one of the basic rules of life: You can't win if you don't play the game.

JOE KNOWS

Football quarterback Joe Montana not only showed up, but consistently demonstrated the drive that made him one of sport's most respected and successful players. While some athletes struggle to maintain their focus and purpose after achieving a career pinnacle like the Super Bowl, Montana's interest and enthusiasm never wavered.

"I felt I had to prove myself every day, every game, every season," Montana said. "When I got to Notre Dame, nothing I had done at Ringgold High in Monongahela, Pennsylvania mattered. When I got to the 49'ers, nothing I had done at Notre Dame mattered. And when I got to Kansas City, nothing I had done in San Francisco mattered."

MOTIVATION MATTERS

In a 1992 *USA Today* survey, 805 American adults were asked, "What caused you to stop dieting before losing all the weight you wanted?" The top two reasons? 39% said they got "discouraged"; 24% cited a "lack of interest."

Remember: The more enthused, the more you lose!

Lean *for* Life®
DAILY ACTION PLAN

Week _____ **Day** _____ **Date** _____

Time	Meal Plans	Serving Size	Carbs (grams)
_____	**Breakfast**		
	Protein		
	Fruit or grain		
	Beverage		
_____	**Protein Snack**		
_____	**Lunch**		
	Protein		
	Vegetable		
	Lettuce		
	Fruit		
	Beverage		
	Miscellaneous		
_____	**Protein Snack**		
_____	**Dinner**		
	Protein		
	Vegetable		
	Lettuce		
	Fruit		
	Beverage		
	Miscellaneous		
_____	**Protein Snack**		
		TOTAL	

Keto Reading _____
Weight _____
Vitamins   AM   Noon   PM
Water _____

Activities _____
_____
_____
_____

Pedometer Steps _____

WEEKLY BODY MEASUREMENTS

Chest _____   Hips _____
Waist _____   Thighs _____
Abdomen _____

SUCCESS LEARNING TOOLS

Read pages # _____
Audio Tape _____
Video _____
CD-ROM _____
Bio-Card™ _____
Affirmation _____

Other _____
Plan to Overcome Today's Obstacles: _____
_____
_____
_____
_____

Notes: _____
_____
_____
_____
_____
_____

CHOOSE ONE DAY EACH WEEK AS YOUR "PROTEIN DAY."

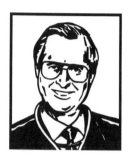

DR. STAMPER

"Motivation is a
decision. Remind
yourself several
times every day
why you've decided
to become
Lean for Life."

Long after Montana had anything to prove to his team, his fans, or himself, he continued to demonstrate remarkable motivation and commitment. He was, above all else, consistent.

It's not enough to be interested and enthusiastic about your program *part of the time.* As you begin your second week of "Phase 1: Weight Loss," remember that *consistency counts.*

HEMINGWAY'S CONSISTENT WAYS

After interviewing writer Ernest Hemingway for *The Paris Review* in 1958, George Plimpton noted: "He keeps track of his daily progress— 'so as not to kid myself'—on a large chart made out of the side of a cardboard packing case and set up against the wall under the nose of a mounted gazelle head. The numbers on the chart showing the daily output of words differ from 450, 575, 462, 1250, back to 512, the higher figures on days Hemingway puts in extra work so he won't feel guilty spending the following days fishing on the Gulf Stream."

Though Hemingway wrote nine novels and nearly 70 short stories, he was not a prolific writer. He was, however, disciplined and consistent, producing an average of two pages a day. His strategy: "Work every day. No matter what has happened the day or night before, get up and bite on the nail."

There will always be plenty of reasons why you can't, won't, or shouldn't eat well or exercise on a given day. Your challenge is to decide if you'll give those excuses enough power to derail your dream or whether you'll "bite on the nail" and stay committed enough, consistently enough, to really do it—day in and day out, no matter what.

"MR. MITO" SAYS:

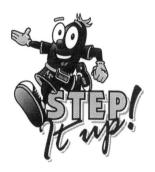

"Be sure to increase your level of activity enthusiastically but gradually. If you don't increase, you won't enjoy the benefits. If you do too much too soon, you run the risk of becoming sore, fatigued, or injured. So step to it—but don't push it!"

ANY QUESTIONS?

Q: *I've noticed that sometimes my breath smells and my mouth tastes bad. What's going on?*

A: Ketones are excreted through the lungs as well as the kidneys. This accounts for the "keto-odor" some people occasionally notice. Make a point to brush your teeth regularly to keep your mouth fresh and clean. You might also try calorie-free breath fresheners between meals.

Q: *Why can't I just eat frozen diet meals from my supermarket?*

A: They tend to be too low in protein and too high in calories, carbohydrates, and fat.

Your Turn

Ten days ago, you listed your reasons for becoming Lean for Life on notecards. Take a minute to review your list. Choose any one of your reasons and declare it again in writing:

"I'm learning to become Lean for Life because _____

_____

_____

_____ ."

After you write it down, read it out loud. This may feel a little silly at first, but revisiting your reasons is an effective way to reinforce your enthusiasm, confidence, and optimism.

Each day is a new beginning. You have good reasons to drop bad habits and stay focused on what really matters to you. This exercise is a way to start each day by celebrating your decision!

DAY 9

BIOMODIFIERS™

You can do things that will make it easier for your body to lose weight.

You've already taken two vital steps toward losing weight. You're eating foods that are high in protein and low in fat, calories, and carbohydrates. You're also exercising gently. And it's working. In just nine days, you're already seeing—and feeling—results.

You're also making progress in other ways that are much less obvious. Right this minute—as you read this page—your body and mind are working together to regulate your body and create your mental state. What we've learned from our patients, and what researchers are beginning to more fully understand, is that any given task is easier to perform when you are in a particular mental state appropriate to that task.

Like most people, you probably learn best when you're relaxed and alert. But let's say you're in a situation where you need to learn something new but you're tense and tired. What can you do about it? You can change your sluggish, grumpy mental state into a relaxed, alert mental state *on purpose*. You may already be familiar with the concept of behavior modification, also known as Behavior Mod—learning to replace non-productive behaviors with behaviors that help you achieve the results you desire, such as a better job, a happier child, or a leaner, healthier body.

At Lindora, we teach a concept we call *BioModification*,™ also known as *BioMod*.™ With BioMod, you can learn to change your biochemistry and therefore your mental state from one that is *less* productive to one that is *more* productive. That's right! You can learn how to modify your mental state at will. We call this activity or experience a *BioModifier.*

People have much greater control over their mental states than previously believed. At Lindora, we had an inkling this was true in the early days when we installed "skinny mirrors" in our clinics as a way of helping patients appreciate the fact that a thinner, healthier body was possible. When patients looked into the mirrors and saw a thinner version of themselves, it helped their brains become more comfortable with the change even before it became a reality.

For many years, Dr. Stamper has also encouraged patients to cultivate what he calls an "inner smile." He counsels people who are experiencing frustration on the program to pause, take a deep breath, hold it briefly, and then visualize an internal smile as they exhale. Our patients who regularly do this report an immediate change in attitude.

Over the years, our understanding of the mind-body connection has deepened. It's clearer than ever that you can intentionally affect your mind and emotions. Through your actions you can create conditions that change your brain chemistry, and therefore change your mental state, in ways that make it easier for you to accomplish a specific purpose, such as achieving and maintaining lean weight.

A BioModifier is an experience or activity that changes what's going on in your brain. Sometimes what goes on in your brain primarily affects your mental state, and sometimes what goes on in your brain primarily affects your physical body. Sleeping, exercising, sitting in the sunshine, listening to music—these are all physical BioModifiers. Mental training techniques such as positive affirmations, mental rehearsal, and brief visualizations are mental BioModifiers.

You've already begun using a number of BioModifiers. Ketosis and exercise are examples of physical BioModifiers. By being in ketosis, for example, you're directing your brain to signal the body to increase its fat-burning capacity. By regularly engaging in gentle exercise, you stimulate your brain's ability to produce "feel-good" chemicals such as endorphins (at Lindora we call them "Lindorphins") and signal your muscle cells to make structural changes that increase fat-burning and carbohydrate metabolism.

You may also recognize that you're learning to use a number of mental BioModifiers. You're learning how to replace negative self-talk

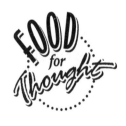

"Success is living the life you want."

— Christopher Morley

Lean *for* Life®
DAILY ACTION PLAN

Week _____ Day _____ Date _____

Time	Meal Plans	Serving Size	Carbs (grams)
	Breakfast		
	Protein		
	Fruit or grain		
	Beverage		
	Protein Snack		
	Lunch		
	Protein		
	Vegetable		
	Lettuce		
	Fruit		
	Beverage		
	Miscellaneous		
	Protein Snack		
	Dinner		
	Protein		
	Vegetable		
	Lettuce		
	Fruit		
	Beverage		
	Miscellaneous		
	Protein Snack		
	TOTAL		

Keto Reading _____

Weight _____

Vitamins   AM   Noon   PM

Water _____

Activities _____

_____

_____

Pedometer Steps _____

WEEKLY BODY MEASUREMENTS

Chest _____   Hips _____

Waist _____   Thighs _____

Abdomen _____

SUCCESS LEARNING TOOLS

Read pages # _____

Audio Tape _____

Video _____

CD-ROM _____

Bio-Card™ _____

Affirmation _____

_____

Other _____

Plan to Overcome Today's Obstacles:

_____

_____

_____

_____

Notes: _____

_____

_____

_____

_____

CHOOSE ONE DAY EACH WEEK AS YOUR "PROTEIN DAY."

with positive images and messages that you are putting in place on purpose. In the days ahead you'll be learning how to use additional BioModifiers to increase your range of options.

Your mind and body are already on your side. They're working hard to help. Once you begin regularly relying on BioModifiers, it will become even easier to achieve your goal.

Your Turn

BioModifiers are things we do to help ourselves get what we want by changing what's happening in our brains and in our bodies.

What would happen if you were to give yourself permission to spend five minutes doing any of the following BioModifiers?

❑ Touch, love, and talk to your dog or cat.

❑ Take a five-minute nap.

❑ Daydream in a safe, loving place where you're completely at peace.

❑ Polish a ring or a piece of silver that has value to you.

❑ Read your favorite poem and allow yourself to absorb its form and meaning.

❑ Laugh! Call your funniest friend for a chat. Flip on the TV and watch a few minutes of your favorite old sit-coms.

❑ Enjoy looking at photographs of people you love.

❑ Put on some music and dance.

Does it work? Why not try it and find out?

WHAT DOROTHY KNOWS

Upon entering our clinics, visitors pass a wall plaque that reads "Lindora Medical Clinics: Comprehensive Weight Control." We've always thought that was a perfect description of the work we do. But if Dorothy, a 48-year-old university administrator from Los Angeles, had her way, the signs would read "Comprehensive *Life* Control."

I met Dorothy one afternoon while visiting our Westwood clinic, just a short walk from Dorothy's office on the UCLA campus. She had lost 45 pounds on the program three years earlier and had regained 10 of them over the previous six months. During that period, she explained, her life had become chaotic. She ended a long-term relationship, moved into a new home, and had been under enormous pressure at work.

"The real reason I decided to do the program again wasn't to lose the 10 pounds as much as it was to regain a sense of balance and control in my life," Dorothy explained. "When I did it the first time, I felt an incredible sense of power and purpose that spilled over into everything I did. I cultivated what I call 'life skills.' When I realized some of those skills were becoming rusty, I knew it was time for a tune-up."

Our conversation made my day. Dorothy is one of those people I think of as "daily heroes." She identifed a problem, rallied her resources, and developed a plan of action. She went for it. Rather than perceiving her weight gain as a catastrophe, she chose to view it as a "wake-up call," an opportunity to refine her skills and get back in control.

When I talked with the manager of our Westwood clinic several weeks later, she mentioned that Dorothy had succeeded in losing the 10 pounds she'd regained.

I wasn't a bit surprised.

YOU ARE WHAT YOU THINK

*You can learn to use your thoughts and
feelings to achieve what you want.*

"Why do I even try? Every time I lose weight, I gain it back—
and then some."

"This one piece won't hurt. And besides, who will know?"

"If I lose too much weight, I'm going to have to buy new clothes. I
don't have the money or the time to shop."

"My whole family is fat. What makes me think I can be different?"

Negative thoughts like these seriously undermine your efforts to
lose weight. That's why we say that to change your body, you have to
change your mind.

Each of us responds to events in our lives according to how we
understand and interpret what is happening to us. If our brain tells us
something is dangerous, we respond one way. When it tells us
something is difficult, we respond in another. And if our brain says,
"This is a worthwhile challenge and you can succeed" our response is
quite different.

Let's say you're meeting a friend for lunch at an Italian restaurant
known for its three-cheese manicotti. You plan to order broiled fish and
steamed vegetables. If you say to yourself, "I feel good about this plan.

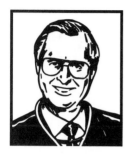

DR. STAMPER

"Make sure you take at least 20 minutes to eat a meal. It takes that long for your stomach to tell your brain it's full."

The food will be delicious and I'll feel satisfied. I know I can do this," chances are you'll be right. You *will* be able to do it and you *will* feel good about it.

On the other hand, let's say you're feeling sorry for yourself. If you're thinking: "Why do I always have to suffer? I don't get to eat out that often. I don't think I'll be able to do it. My willpower is shot," it's a safe bet you *won't* be able to do it and you *won't* feel good about it.

Call it the power of expectation. If you expect the worst, you're more likely to get it. If self-defeating thoughts are swirling around in your head, the results you'll get are likely to be negative. The goal, of course, is to change the outcome by changing the way you react in such situations. How you *choose* to experience an event, person, place, or circumstance affects how you experience it.

If you find that negative thoughts sometimes get in your way, these success strategies can help:

1. *Listen to yourself.* Become more sensitive to your thoughts and feelings. Realize which negative messages get triggered and under what circumstances. To be successful, you need to develop different habits and skills. One of the most important is self-awareness.

2. *Replace negative thoughts and statements with positive ones.* As soon as you hear a harmful, negative message, pause and replace it with a positive one. This may sound contrived at first, but it begins to feel natural the more you do it.

   Does this mean that you tell yourself you look forward to exercise when you don't? Absolutely! You can say something like, "I love the way my body and muscles feel after I exercise. I sleep better at night and have more energy during the day." Whatever words you choose, you can counter the negative with something positive right on the spot.

   Maria, who is 18 pounds away from her weight-loss goal of 86 pounds, refers to her trips to the gym as "traveling." When friends invite her to dinner, she says, "Sorry, can't tonight. I'm traveling to Italy." She loves saying it—and it reminds her of the reward she's promised herself once she achieves her goal.

3. *Practice.* Successful weight loss involves *consistently* replacing negative old patterns with positive new ones. To truly break old habits, it's important to practice the new ones again and again. "Once in a while" or "every now and then" won't cut it.

   Mental training techniques, which we'll discuss in more detail on Day 16, provide an opportunity to rehearse and practice positive patterns in your mind hundreds of times. This consistent repetition has a powerful influence and can lead to lasting change. Negative patterns of thought wither and stronger patterns of self-respect and self-confidence take their place.

This program is not just about how to lose weight and keep it off. One of our guiding principles is to teach you—and then remind you—that you always have *choices* and *options*. You can decide what to eat and what not to eat. And most important of all: You can decide what to think and what not to think.

The choices you make directly impact the results you get.

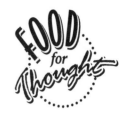

"Our life is what our thoughts make it."

— Marcus Aurelius

PARTY PLANNING

Life doesn't screech to a halt just because you've decided to lose weight. During the next several weeks, it's possible that you'll be attending a party, reception, or special event. They can be fun, but they can also be a minefield of temptation. One way to maintain your motivation is to plan ahead. These tips will help:

❑ *Nix the alcohol.* Alcohol packs a wicked triple punch. It contains empty calories. It impairs judgment and lowers your resistance to impulse eating. Alcohol also interferes with your body's ability to burn stored fat for fuel. Stick with caffeine-free diet soda or mineral water with a slice of lemon or lime.

❑ *Steer clear of buffets and party platters.* Out of sight doesn't necessarily mean out of mind, but it's a lot easier to resist that homemade potato salad or those gourmet cookies when they're on the other side of the room.

❑ *Eat before you go.* You'll find it easier to resist temptation if you're full.

❑ *Be up front.* If you're invited to a dinner party and know the host or hostess well, explain in advance that you're on the program. Ask what is being served or offer to bring something you know you can eat. You're likely to find that your host will be supportive and willing to accommodate you.

❑ *Pack protein.* Take a couple of protein supplements with you so you always have options.

Remember: Being a guest at a party, reception, or event isn't about food—it's about good times, good conversation, and good friends.

Lean *for* Life®
DAILY ACTION PLAN

Week _____ **Day** _____ **Date** _____

Time	Meal Plans	Serving Size	Carbs (grams)
_____	**Breakfast**		
	Protein		
	Fruit or grain		
	Beverage		
_____	**Protein Snack**		
_____	**Lunch**		
	Protein		
	Vegetable		
	Lettuce		
	Fruit		
	Beverage		
	Miscellaneous		
_____	**Protein Snack**		
_____	**Dinner**		
	Protein		
	Vegetable		
	Lettuce		
	Fruit		
	Beverage		
	Miscellaneous		
_____	**Protein Snack**		
		TOTAL	

Keto Reading _____

Weight _____

Vitamins   AM   Noon   PM

Water _____

Activities _____
_____
_____

Pedometer Steps _____

WEEKLY BODY MEASUREMENTS

Chest _____   Hips _____

Waist _____   Thighs _____

Abdomen _____

SUCCESS LEARNING TOOLS

Read pages # _____

Audio Tape _____

Video _____

CD-ROM _____

Bio-Card™ _____

Affirmation _____
_____

Other _____

Plan to Overcome Today's Obstacles:
_____
_____
_____
_____
_____

Notes:
_____
_____
_____
_____
_____

CHOOSE ONE DAY EACH WEEK AS YOUR "PROTEIN DAY."

AFFIRMING THE POSITIVE

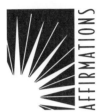

AFFIRMATIONS

Over the next 10 days, you'll have a unique opportunity to use, think about, and react to *affirmations*. Affirmations are a form of mental rehearsal that can help you set goals, make choices, and implement new patterns of thinking and behaving.

On Day 20, we'll take a closer look at how affirmations work as BioModifiers, why they're effective, and how you can benefit from using them. Between now and then, make a point of reading the affirmations featured each day. Write them down every day on your Daily Action Plan. Say them out loud. Repeat them. Think about them. Notice your reactions.

Today's affirmation:

"I am enjoying reminding myself that I am worthy of love and respect."

DAY 11

LEARN TO MANAGE STRESS AND YOU'LL LEARN TO MANAGE FOOD

You can learn healthy new ways to manage your stress and anxiety.

Stress and food. In the grand scheme of great combinations, they rank right up there with Lucy and Ricky or fireworks and the Fourth of July. If you consider how *often* and how *automatically* we rely on food to manage our anxiety, medicate our feelings, and manipulate our moods, the link between the two is undeniable.

We've grown up in a culture in which food is much more than a source of fuel. It symbolizes a spectrum of human needs and wants, including comfort, companionship, reward, punishment, escape, control, and power.

As infants, we had bottles shoved in our mouths to relax and quiet us. As kids, we were rewarded for good behavior with cookies and candy. A friend of mine, now 41, still remembers being bribed into behaving during his dental check-ups. Twice a year, his payoff for enduring the drill without a tantrum was a hot fudge sundae on the trip home.

Food—and the withholding of it—has long been used to control children's behavior. Remember the threat of all threats: being sent to

Lean *for* Life®
DAILY ACTION PLAN

Week _____ Day _____ Date _____

Time	Meal Plans	Serving Size	Carbs (grams)
	Breakfast		
	Protein		
	Fruit or grain		
	Beverage		
	Protein Snack		
	Lunch		
	Protein		
	Vegetable		
	Lettuce		
	Fruit		
	Beverage		
	Miscellaneous		
	Protein Snack		
	Dinner		
	Protein		
	Vegetable		
	Lettuce		
	Fruit		
	Beverage		
	Miscellaneous		
	Protein Snack		
		TOTAL	

Keto Reading _____
Weight _____
Vitamins   AM   Noon   PM
Water _____

Activities _____
_____
_____
_____

Pedometer Steps _____

WEEKLY BODY MEASUREMENTS
Chest _____   Hips _____
Waist _____   Thighs _____
Abdomen _____

SUCCESS LEARNING TOOLS
Read pages # _____
Audio Tape _____
Video _____
CD-ROM _____
Bio-Card ™ _____
Affirmation _____

Other _____
Plan to Overcome Today's Obstacles: _____
_____
_____
_____
_____

Notes: _____
_____
_____
_____
_____

CHOOSE ONE DAY EACH WEEK AS YOUR "PROTEIN DAY."

bed without supper? Even Beaver Cleaver heard that one. And how many times was dessert the reward for cleaning your plate, even if it meant eating more than you wanted or needed?

When you look at how we've been culturally conditioned to think about and use food, it's no surprise so many of us have grown up relying on it to cope with the stress and anxiety of our everyday lives.

There are, however, a number of healthier, more effective ways to address stress. Throughout this book, you'll find suggestions for effective problem-solving strategies, mental training, and breathing exercises. Let's take a look at one of the most effective stress-reducers you can treat yourself to. It's fast, free, and easy to do. What's more, it feels terrific and offers lasting benefits.

When you're "stressed out," where do you typically feel the tension first? For most of us, stiffness and tenderness in the neck and shoulders are dead giveaways that all is not well. Rather than medicate or mask the tension by crunching potato chips or chewing cookies, try a more active, hands-on approach.

Begin by reaching up with both hands to the base of your skull, one hand under each ear. Feel the muscles and the bones. (It's only fair to warn you up front—if you're doing it correctly, it's going to be uncomfortable at first.) Press firmly against the bone without loosening the pressure and move your hands gently back and forth so

Another Lean for Life Success Story

"I spent the first 32 years of my life using food to numb my feelings and manage my stress. I grew up in a home where sweets were my mother's solution to every problem. When I was 14, a kid I had a crush on invited my best friend to the Halloween dance. That night, my mother made me a pineapple upside-down cake. I ate the whole thing. It wasn't until I started the program that I realized how a pattern established years ago was still taking its toll. Now, rather than reaching for food whenever I'm stressed, I stop and ask myself, 'What do I really want? What do I really need?'"

—Jessica

that you cover the entire width and length of the muscle. Hold this as tightly as you can, reminding yourself that while any discomfort you may experience is temporary, the results will be long lasting.

When you first begin doing this, make a point to apply at least one minute of uninterrupted pressure. It takes that long to begin relaxing muscle tension. After a minute or so, the pain will begin to lessen and you'll know you're doing it correctly. Continue rubbing for at least another two to four minutes.

The more you rub, the less it will hurt. Rub from the base of your skull under your ears, down the sides of your neck, and out to your shoulder blades. Repeat this several times a day to prevent the tension from recurring.

The second day you do this, expect your neck and shoulders to be tender. They may even feel bruised. Whatever you do, don't let this slow you down. This is a natural result of having worked acidic muscles so vigorously the day before. If you allow too much time to pass between rubdowns, the neck and shoulder muscles will tighten back up and you'll have to start all over again. Begin gently until it starts feeling more comfortable, than do it as vigorously as you can.

Continue this process daily. Within four to seven days, you'll find that your neck and shoulder muscles are much less tense. You'll want to give yourself a quick check-up a couple of times a week. Reach beneath the base of the skull and about the middle of the neck and press firmly. If you don't experience any significant tenderness, your neck and shoulders are tension free. If you do locate a trigger point that hurts—and sooner or later, you're bound to—massage it away.

This active approach eases away stress symptoms. Give it a chance to work for you. It's a perfect example of how your health—and your ability to enhance it—is truly in your hands.

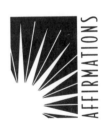

AFFIRMATIONS

"I feel good about choosing foods that nourish me and keep me healthy."

"KETO-CONSISTENCY" COUNTS

Consistency is one of the "secrets" of success on this program. Once you're in ketosis, stay there. Why make "Phase 1: Weight Loss" more challenging than it needs to be? If you discover you're not in ketosis, review your previous day's Action Plan to see where the excess carbohydrates came from. Then take action!

Your Turn

What causes you stress? By identifying the people, places, events, and circumstances that cause stress in your life, you will become more aware of how your stress can influence *what* you eat, *when* you eat, and *how often* you eat.

Put a mark next to the statements that you generally find to be true:

❑   My work is too demanding.

❑   I don't like my job.

❑   My family responsibilities often feel overwhelming.

❑   I'm self-conscious about my appearance and/or concerned about my weight.

❑   I don't have enough fun or "down time" to do what I want.

❑   I worry about my personal safety.

❑   I've been divorced or separated within the last year.

❑   Someone I care about has been ill or has died within the last year.

❑   I'm concerned about my job security.

❑   I worry about my health.

❑   I have difficulty communicating with my boss and/or co-workers.

❑   I'm fighting regularly with a relative or friend.

❑   My income is too low to meet my monthly bills.

❑   I became a parent within the last year.

❑   I am a care-giver to a family member or friend.

❑   I recently made a large purchase (house, car, tuition).

❑   I've moved within the last year.

❑   I'm concerned about my level of physical fitness.

List any other ongoing or major causes of stress in your life:

_____

_____

_____

HOW DO YOU REACT–AND RESPOND–TO STRESS?

Now that you've identified your major sources of stress, let's look at how you respond. What impact does stress have on your body, your brain, and your behavior? Review the following list. Circle 0 for never, 1 for sometimes, and 2 for always.

I notice the following physical responses to stress:

0	1	2	headaches
0	1	2	change in attitude
0	1	2	fatigue
0	1	2	interrupted sleep/sleeping too much
0	1	2	indigestion
0	1	2	sore back and/or shoulder muscles

In my behavior, I notice:

0	1	2	decreased productivity
0	1	2	increased irritability and anger
0	1	2	increased eating and snacking
0	1	2	increased smoking
0	1	2	increased drug or alcohol intake
0	1	2	increased spending
0	1	2	withdrawal and a desire not to be bothered by others

I notice the following psychological responses to stress:

0	1	2	sadness or depression
0	1	2	difficulty concentrating
0	1	2	feeling emotionally drained
0	1	2	feeling impulsive
0	1	2	forgetfulness
0	1	2	a desire to eat more
0	1	2	feeling anxious or short-tempered

The more 2's you've circled, the more attention you need to pay to how you manage your stress.

Over the next several days, notice how you respond to stress. Do you eat more than you want or need? Consider how BioModifiers (review Day 9) can help change the signal you're sending your brain from "Eat!" to "Let's do something positive."

ANY QUESTIONS?

Q: *I love walking for a few minutes, but I get bored easily. Any suggestions?*

A: Do you ever use a stereo headset while walking? Time flies when you listen to talk radio, books on tape, or your favorite music. You might also invite a friend, neighbor, or family member to join you.

Make a point to include a variety of activities in your weekly schedule. Go bicycling. Try the stair climbing, rowing, or cross-country ski machines at your gym. Dance to your favorite music—even if it's alone in your living room. Whatever you do, remember to do it *gently*.

These kinds of activities will help you avoid falling into a rut. They'll also reduce the risk of injury or quitting the program that can come from using the same muscles in the same way every day.

WHO'S IN CHARGE OF YOUR "INNER COMMITTEE"?

You will learn how your "inner voices" compete for your attention.

Grace is an accomplished artist. In recent years, she has earned a national reputation for her dramatic murals. Her work is featured in top galleries and her first one-woman exhibit opened to rave reviews. Yet there are days when Grace wakes up feeling like a fraud, wondering when the world will discover she has no talent.

A.J. is the most outgoing, fun-loving character in his fraternity. He's a practical joker with an offbeat sense of humor and a magnetic personality. There are days, however, when the thought of interacting with people makes A.J. cringe. He retreats to his bedroom, unplugs his phone, and listens to music for hours at a time.

Monica is ecstatic about her weight-loss success. She's lost 27 pounds and is more than halfway to her goal. But there are times, she admits, when she finds herself questioning whether her goal is "really worth the effort" and whether she has "whatever it takes" to maintain her weight loss.

Like Grace, A.J., and Monica, we all experience an array of contradictory emotions that influence how we think, act, and feel.

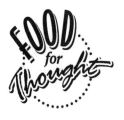

"We ask ourselves,

who am I to be

brilliant, gorgeous,

talented, and

fabulous? Actually,

who are you

not to be?"

— Marianne Williamson

Within each of us exists an "Inner Committee" of conflicting voices competing to be heard. One of your inner voices is loving and supportive. Another is harsh and critical. There's a frightened one, a joyful one, and an angry one. There's even a curious, playful one.

While each of these inner voices has a point of view and an agenda, you are ultimately the "chairperson" of your Inner Committee. Every thinking, responsible person has moments when "I can't" or "I won't" messages threaten to limit his or her options. By strengthening the positive inner voices that are open, loving, and supportive, you can free yourself to move forward and manage your moments of self-doubt more effectively.

Until you understand how this chorus of inner voices works, it's easy to feel confused. But once you do, you can learn to rely on your Inner Committee to help you zero in on what's really important to you.

Perhaps you can recognize some or all of these common voices, as well as adding several of your own:

Your Frightened Voice "I'm afraid I'm not going to do this right."

Your Angry Voice "I'm never allowed to do or say what I want!"

Your Critical Voice "Don't even bother— you don't deserve it."

Your Joyful Voice "Hey, let's do this! This is wonderful!"

Your Curious Voice "I'll figure out a way to do this!"

Your Loving Voice "I'm with you—no matter what!"

Your Confident Voice "I can do it!"

Considering the various voices vying for power and control, it's no wonder we sometimes feel or think one thing today, only to feel or think something quite different tomorrow. Understanding these apparent contradictions can help you develop a balanced perspective on your inner conflicts. It can also remind you that whatever voice is speaking at the moment isn't the only voice with something to say.

There are times when one of your voices may sound especially shrill, obnoxious, or destructive. It's important to listen to all of them, not only those that are pleasant and encouraging. The voices that are afraid or angry often perform an important service in alerting us to be cautious.

Lean *for* Life®
DAILY ACTION PLAN

Week _____ Day _____ Date _____

Time	Meal Plans	Serving Size	Carbs (grams)
	Breakfast		
	Protein		
	Fruit or grain		
	Beverage		
	Protein Snack		
	Lunch		
	Protein		
	Vegetable		
	Lettuce		
	Fruit		
	Beverage		
	Miscellaneous		
	Protein Snack		
	Dinner		
	Protein		
	Vegetable		
	Lettuce		
	Fruit		
	Beverage		
	Miscellaneous		
	Protein Snack		
	TOTAL		

Keto Reading _____
Weight _____
Vitamins   AM   Noon   PM
Water _____

Activities _____
_____
_____
_____

Pedometer Steps _____

WEEKLY BODY MEASUREMENTS
Chest _____   Hips _____
Waist _____   Thighs _____
Abdomen _____

SUCCESS LEARNING TOOLS
Read pages # _____
Audio Tape _____
Video _____
CD-ROM _____
Bio-Card ™ _____
Affirmation _____

Other _____
Plan to Overcome Today's Obstacles:
_____
_____
_____
_____
_____

Notes: _____
_____
_____

CHOOSE ONE DAY EACH WEEK AS YOUR "PROTEIN DAY."

DEALING WITH SELF-DOUBT

What do you do when you hear your Critical Voice, the one that says: "I know myself—I'll do fine on this program for a while, then I'll put all the weight right back on"?

For starters, you want to recognize it and respond as the adult in charge, perhaps with something as simple as, "I choose to ignore what you're saying right now and continue my weight-loss plans." In addition, you also want to do everything you can to strengthen the powerful, positive voice that knows you will be successful. This requires setting aside some time every day for mental training practice, just as you would for physical exercise. This needs to be protected time when you know you won't be interrupted.

You can also "sit in" on a meeting of your Inner Committee. Write down what your different voices are saying, as well as your response to them. Make note of the negative comments you're hearing, but focus primarily on what your loving, joyful, curious, confident voices say to counter negative messages. Cultivate strong positive voices so that they can overpower the negative ones.

Let's say, for example, you're beginning to notice changes in how you look and feel. While part of you will be thrilled and think, "I knew you could do it!" there may also be a part that's terrified by your progress. You may hear an antagonistic voice—perhaps a combination of your Frightened Voice ("I'm afraid I'm not going to do this right") and your Critical Voice ("Don't even bother—you don't deserve it!").

When most of us hear our negative inner voices, our first inclination is to silence or ignore them. There is, however, another possibility. Whenever you become aware of a negative voice, you can welcome the fact that you're being warned of possible self-sabotage. Listen carefully to what the voice is saying. Is it telling you something you need to hear? If it's simply afraid and reflecting old doubts, reassure it. Tell yourself it will be okay, just as you would tell a child in need of comfort. Then do what you've decided is in your best interest.

Remember: The members of your Inner Committee aren't issuing commands. They're merely voicing fears and concerns. The decision as to which voice has the greater influence is ultimately yours.

Your Turn

Since you began your program, it's a safe bet the voices that populate your Inner Committee have each had something to say. Which have the greatest power? Which seem most persistent? Write down a message that each of your inner voices has sent since you started the program.

Your Frightened Voice "_____"

Your Angry Voice "_____"

Your Critical Voice "_____"

Your Joyful Voice "_____"

Your Curious Voice "_____"

Your Loving Voice "_____"

Your Confident Voice "_____"

Another Lean for Life Success Story

"I know it sounds weird, but I visualize the Seven Dwarfs when I think of my Inner Committee. Before I started the program, Grumpy had a lot of power. So did Bashful. I always listened to the inner voice that told me not to take risks or try anything new. Now that I've lost 26 pounds, I hear a lot more from Happy. Grumpy and Bashful still try to exert their influence, but I remind myself that they only have as much power as I give them. How I choose to feel—and what I choose to do—is totally up to me."

— *Kyle*

Then & Now

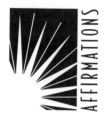

"I am worthy
of love
and respect."

ANY QUESTIONS?

Q: *Even when I'm in ketosis, my ketostick never turns dark purple. Why not?*

A: The color on your ketostick can be influenced by a number of factors. Some people never have a dark purple ketostick because of individual variations in their body's physiology. If you make a diet error and eat too many carbohydrates, your body won't be burning fat, you won't be in ketosis, and you won't have color on your ketostick. On "Phase 1: Weight Loss" menu days, your ketostick will typically show a lighter color than on Protein Days because your menu includes more carbohydrates.

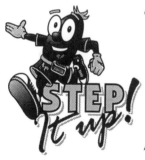

"MR. MITO" SAYS:

"The New England Journal of Medicine reports that people tend to overestimate their level of activity while underestimating their food intake. That's why it's so important to accurately and consistently fill out your Daily Action Plan. How are you doing with yours?"

TURNING OBSTACLES INTO OPPORTUNITIES

You can learn how to see problems as possibilities for personal growth—and you can become more skilled at solving them.

Amelia Earhart. Jackie Robinson. Michelangelo Buonarroti. Barbara Jordan. Dr. Jonas Salk. Helen Keller. Thomas Edison. Wolfgang Amadeus Mozart.

These extraordinary achievers have more in common than a place in the history books. Every one of them faced—and overcame—tremendous obstacles in order to make their mark in the world. Yet as unique as their gifts and achievements were, you can bet they each experienced their share of setbacks, fear, frustration, disappointment, and self-doubt.

Anyone who has ever accomplished anything has encountered challenges along the way. Writer Huston Smith, a student and teacher of the world's great religions, believes that our problems are a gift, an opportunity life offers so that we may make spiritual discoveries. In learning to overcome difficulties, Smith suggests, we learn to search for answers, to struggle with life's greater issues, and to experience growth.

While it's doubtful that most people would think of the obstacles encountered on a weight-loss program as "spiritual," the character traits we develop when we face challenges—patience, insight, vision,

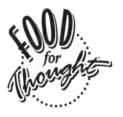

"All things are

difficult before

they are easy."

— Thomas Fuller

focus, and self-respect, among others—can bolster and strengthen our spirit and sense of mastery on this or any other self-improvement pursuit.

Over the past 12 days, it's likely that you've found yourself in situations where you didn't respond as well as you would have liked. Maybe there was a night when your cravings got the best of you. Perhaps you skipped your exercise or decided to "test" the program by seeing whether you could eat your favorite food and still remain in ketosis.

Whatever obstacles you face on this program, remember that you always have a *choice* as to how to react. You can choose to feel bad and give up, or you can use your experience as an opportunity to learn and grow. Your attitude—the mindset with which you approach problems—has a direct impact on your ability to transform obstacles into opportunities.

People who consistently demonstrate this positive "achievement attitude" share three common traits—belief, desire, and persistence:

1. *They believe it's possible to improve their situation.* When you believe that what you do influences the results you get, you will see yourself as someone who can act effectively to get what you want.

2. *They have a genuine desire to improve their situation.* Not everyone wants to improve his or her life. Sometimes we become so comfortable with our problems that they fit like an old slipper. It's hard to give them up. Problems sometimes serve a purpose, such as helping us avoid the challenge of change, or keeping others at a distance. Next time you're grappling with a problem, ask yourself how much you *really* want to solve it. Are there hidden payoffs for *not* overcoming the problem? What, if anything, are you getting out of staying "stuck"?

3. *They are persistent in improving their situation.* A recent article in *Parade* featured women who had beaten enormous odds to achieve greatness. All of them—the college president, the business entreprenuer, the breast-cancer researcher, the naval educator— talked about the importance of tenacity and trying a variety of approaches until one finally worked. They refused to give up. For them, failure was not an option.

As you near the halfway mark of "Phase 1: Weight Loss," ask yourself: "Do I possess an 'achievement attitude?' Do I believe in my ability to accomplish my goal?"

If so, what can you do in the coming weeks to reinforce it? If not, what's stopping you right now from applying what you've learned to transform your obstacles into opportunities?

Lean *for* Life®
DAILY ACTION PLAN

Week _____   Day _____   Date _____

Time	Meal Plans	Serving Size	Carbs (grams)
_____	**Breakfast** _____		
	Protein		
	Fruit or grain		
	Beverage		
	_____		
	_____		
	_____		
_____	**Protein Snack** _____		
_____	**Lunch** _____		
	Protein		
	Vegetable		
	Lettuce		
	Fruit		
	Beverage		
	Miscellaneous		
	_____		
	_____		
_____	**Protein Snack** _____		
_____	**Dinner** _____		
	Protein		
	Vegetable		
	Lettuce		
	Fruit		
	Beverage		
	Miscellaneous		
	_____		
	_____		
_____	**Protein Snack** _____		
		TOTAL	

Keto Reading _____
Weight _____
Vitamins   AM _____   Noon _____   PM _____
Water _____

Activities _____
_____
_____

Pedometer Steps _____

WEEKLY BODY MEASUREMENTS
Chest _____   Hips _____
Waist _____   Thighs _____
Abdomen _____

SUCCESS LEARNING TOOLS
Read pages # _____
Audio Tape _____
Video _____
CD-ROM _____
Bio-Card™ _____
Affirmation _____

Other _____
Plan to Overcome Today's Obstacles:
_____
_____
_____
_____

Notes:
_____
_____
_____

CHOOSE ONE DAY EACH WEEK AS YOUR "PROTEIN DAY."

Your Turn

Write down three goals you've accomplished in the past five years that you're especially proud of:

1. _____

2. _____

3. _____

List three specific skills, abilities, attitudes, or behaviors that contributed to each of those successes:

Goal #1	Goal #2	Goal #3
_____	_____	_____
_____	_____	_____
_____	_____	_____

Review this list. Are you currently using all of the resources that have helped you succeed in the past? If your answer isn't "Yes," consider how you can more effectively support yourself in achieving your goal.

"MR. MITO" SAYS:

"Studies show that people who begin their day with a healthy breakfast are better able to control their calorie intake throughout the rest of the day. In addition to providing energy and nutrition, breakfast also helps moderate appetite, which makes it easier to avoid midday munchies and binges. Breakfast also benefits your brain as well as your body: studies reveal that breakfast-eaters do better on cognitive tests than breakfast-skippers."

THE EXERCISE ADVANTAGE

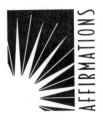

AFFIRMATIONS

Gentle exercise is an investment in your health that:

- ❏ releases tension and promotes relaxation.

- ❏ naturally controls your appetite.

- ❏ accelerates weight loss by increasing mitochondria and burning calories that would otherwise be stored as fat.

- ❏ strengthens your immune system.

- ❏ produces norepinephrine, a chemical that naturally elevates your mood and works as an antidepressant.

- ❏ enhances your overall sense of well-being.

- ❏ tones and firms muscles.

- ❏ helps boost your metabolism.

- ❏ increases your strength and stamina.

- ❏ helps you sleep better.

- ❏ improves your overall flexibility, balance, and coordination.

"I am enjoying doing the things that are helping me become lean and healthy."

DAY
14

PROBLEM SOLVING

You will discover how to solve problems and embrace challenge and change.

Ingrid and Robin are living proof that opposites sometimes attract. They've been best friends since meeting in the second grade nearly 20 years ago. But other than their childhoods and a mutual desire to drop 30 pounds before their upcoming high school reunion, they seem to have little in common.

Ingrid, who recently started her own gourmet catering business, is adventurous, animated, and single. She loves a challenge as much as life itself. Robin, a court reporter who married her college sweetheart five years ago, is much more reserved and conservative. A homebody, she values security and enjoys routine.

Even the way the two friends resolve problems and deal with conflict is as different as night and day. Ingrid considers problems to be an inevitable part of life. She sees them as temporary challenges to be overcome. "You can't have a rainbow," she's fond of saying, "if you don't have the rain."

While Ingrid has always been one to *make* things happen, Robin prefers to *let* things happen. Never one to embrace challenge or change, she procrastinates and passively avoids problems whenever possible.

Robin freely admits that if Ingrid hadn't prodded her to do the Lean for Life program with her, she probably would "never have gotten around to it."

WHAT'S YOUR PROBLEM-SOLVING STYLE?

Ingrid and Robin operate on opposite ends of the problem-solving spectrum. Most of us function somewhere in the middle. We typically welcome some challenges and handle some problems with ease and efficiency, while dodging other challenges and avoiding other problems at all costs.

One of the strongest predictors of success at any endeavor—including weight loss—is one's belief that he or she can solve problems effectively and achieve a desired result. While there's no one "right" way to solve problems or resolve conflicts, this straighforward five-step strategy can be a valuable tool for resolving whatever problems you encounter on your program—and in life:

1. *Identify the problem.* Sounds obvious enough, doesn't it? It is. But sometimes it's so easy to get so wrapped up in how you're reacting to a situation or circumstance that the actual reason you're feeling bad can get lost in the shuffle. Anxiety, uncertainty, anger, depression, disappointment, confusion, guilt, and feelings of inadequacy are all common responses to everyday problems. They aren't, however, the problem itself.

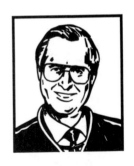

DR. STAMPER

"Food is the most inexpensive, readily available, socially acceptable drug in the world."

REWARD YOURSELF

One great way to stay motivated on the program is to reward yourself as you achieve intermediate goals.

Janet, who is just 12 pounds away from her 50-pound weight-loss goal, treated herself to a manicure when she lost 10 pounds. After she lost 20, she went back for a facial. She celebrated the 30 pound mark by buying a bicycle. And when she celebrates her one-year anniversary, Janet and her best friend plan to celebrate with a ski trip to Lake Tahoe.

How are *you* rewarding yourself? Be sure to celebrate your success along the way. It's a terrific way to stay focused—and to recognize a job well done!

Lean for Life®
DAILY ACTION PLAN

Week _____ Day _____ Date _____

Time	Meal Plans	Serving Size	Carbs (grams)
____	**Breakfast**		
	Protein		
	Fruit or grain		
	Beverage		
____	**Protein Snack**		
____	**Lunch**		
	Protein		
	Vegetable		
	Lettuce		
	Fruit		
	Beverage		
	Miscellaneous		
____	**Protein Snack**		
____	**Dinner**		
	Protein		
	Vegetable		
	Lettuce		
	Fruit		
	Beverage		
	Miscellaneous		
____	**Protein Snack**		
		TOTAL	

Keto Reading _____
Weight _____
Vitamins   AM   Noon   PM
Water _____

Activities _____
_____
_____

Pedometer Steps _____

WEEKLY BODY MEASUREMENTS
Chest _____   Hips _____
Waist _____   Thighs _____
Abdomen _____

SUCCESS LEARNING TOOLS
Read pages # _____
Audio Tape _____
Video _____
CD-ROM _____
Bio-Card™ _____
Affirmation _____
_____

Other _____
Plan to Overcome Today's Obstacles:
_____
_____
_____
_____

Notes: _____
_____
_____
_____
_____
_____

CHOOSE ONE DAY EACH WEEK AS YOUR "PROTEIN DAY."

Ask yourself what's really going on. Rather than reacting or getting caught up in how you're feeling, do your best to objectively identify and define what's truly troubling you. Our patients often find it helpful to write the problem down in a clear, simple sentence. A problem well defined is a problem half solved.

2. *Create a list of possible solutions.* Brainstorm all the ways you can think of to solve the problem. As you write down all the options that come to mind, ignore your critical inner voice, the one that says things like, "That'll never work!"

3. *Choose the best solution.* In many cases, more than one solution will work, yet one is likely to emerge as more effective and productive than the others.

4. *Set realistic goals. You want your goals to be big enough to matter, small enough to achieve, and safe enough to tolerate.* Think of your goal as a dream with a deadline, then make it happen!

    If, for example, your problem is eating too much at night, the solution you came up with may have been to eat a mid-afternoon

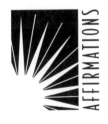

AFFIRMATIONS

"I like seeing myself as an effective problem solver."

Your Turn

It's been two weeks since you first took your measurements. It's time to do it again!

Measure your chest, waist, lower abdomen, hips, and upper thigh, and jot down the numbers below. This is a useful way to keep track of fat loss.

Chest _____   Hips _____

Waist _____   Thigh _____

Abdomen _____

Compare your results with your measurements from "Prep: Day 2." How many total inches have you lost? Where did you lose most?

On Day 28, you'll be comparing your measurements with today's numbers, so keep up the good work!

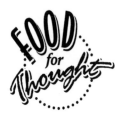

snack so you're not ravenous and out of control. An appropriate goal could be to pack a mid-afternoon snack every morning before leaving for work.

5. *Follow through.* Did you go to the grocery store to buy your snacks? Did you prepare your snack at home so you could take it with you? Did it actually make its way into your purse or briefcase? Last but not least, did you eat your mid-afternoon snack sometime mid-afternoon?

Each of these steps counts. A plan without action is just an idea. You'll find problem-solving easier when you have written down your problem, the solution you've decided to follow, the goals you've set, and the steps needed to achieve the goal.

YOUR PERSONAL SATISFACTION QUOTIENT

How you feel about your life—your work, your family, your relationships, your finances, your health, your body— impacts everything you think, say, and do. Are you physically energetic? Are you happy more often than sad? Do you get along with others? Do you like yourself? Circle the number that reflects how you feel about your life *at this moment:*

| 1 | 2 | 3 | 4 | 5 | 6 | 7 | 8 | 9 | 10 |

I've never been more unhappy.   I'm generally satisfied with my life.   My life is terrific!

You did this exercise on "Prep: Day 2." Refer back to page XX to see whether your answer has changed. If so, what changes does today's score reflect?

5

WEIGHT LOSS
WEEK THREE

DAY 15

VALUES AND VISION

You can create a personal vision that will guide you toward changing your life for the better.

What matters to you? What do you value? How do those values influence your vision of your future?

While these may not be questions you often ask yourself, the answers are reflected every day in the way you live. Your values—the basic principles you live by—directly affect your behavior and decisions. They also influence what you expect and what you'll accept.

What follows is a powerful exercise that has transformed lives. It can help you clarify your values and declare your vision in a way that can provide direction and purpose. The power of this exercise is that it lets you experience yourself—in your imagination—*already being the person you want to be*, having already overcome whatever obstacles await you. *You get to experience yourself already enjoying success, even before the actual changes have taken place.*

During this exercise, you're likely to discover things about yourself that your rational, logical mind might not have noticed before. It may be the first time you've ever seriously questioned what really matters to you.

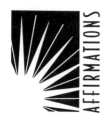

AFFIRMATIONS

"I am enjoying my

gentle exercise."

HOW TO CREATE YOUR VISION STATEMENT

To get the most out of this experience, do it when you're feeling relaxed and receptive. Set aside at least 20 minutes and choose a setting that feels comfortable.

Read the narrative in the "Your Turn" box on page 135 several times. When you come to the passage that invites you to experience yourself saying, "This is what I have, this is what I'm doing as part of my daily life, this is who I am," close your eyes and let yourself enjoy this richly satisfying process.

Take the time to fully experience every part of this vision, adding all the sensory details you can. The more completely you enter into your vision, taking time to experience the scene and the feelings it generates, the more of a guide and an inspiration your vision will be.

THE NEXT STEP

After you've reflected on your vision, write it out in as much detail as you can. What does your life look and feel like? Who are you? How is the person in your vision different from who you are now? Who is sharing it all with you?

Once you've finished, take a few minutes to reread it and fully appreciate what you have created. It's a precious document that clarifies your goals and expectations, who you are, and what's truly important to you.

It's a roadmap to your future.

Another Lean for Life Success Story

"I just sort of took life as it came until the day I did my Vision Statement. It was a real wake-up call. It forced me to take an honest look at what I was—and wasn't—doing to create the healthy, independent lifestyle I always said I wanted. Since I completed the Lean for Life program nine months ago, I've maintained a 42-pound weight loss and enrolled in school to become a massage therapist. It's not always easy, but I have a sense of pride and purpose I never felt before. It feels terrific."

— Gwen

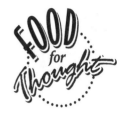

MY VISION STATEMENT

I am waking up in the morning... I'm excited about being alive, excited about the things I will be doing today.

At this moment, I have no need to hurry. I look out the window and see that the sky is crystal clear and beautiful.

I stretch and smile. I let myself become aware of the gifts I've been given... aware of the work I've done... of what I've accomplished... of what I have now... of what I'm doing in my daily life... of who I am. This feels exactly right! I have so much to be grateful for.

This is what I have, this is what I am doing as part of my daily life, this is who I am:

_____

_____

_____

_____

_____

_____

_____

I feel satisfaction in knowing that I am doing what is important to me. I live with a feeling of accomplishment and with a deep sense of inner peace.

My life is full and I feel very much alive. I'm committed to continuing to do the things that help me take care of myself physically, emotionally, intellectually, spiritually, and in every other way.

I'm feeling safe, strong and comfortable. It feels good to know that I deserve all this, and that I'm doing what is important to me.

"You gain strength, courage, and confidence by every experience in which you really stop to look fear in the face. You must do the things you cannot do."

—Eleanor Roosevelt

Lean *for* Life®
DAILY ACTION PLAN

Week _____ Day _____ Date _____

Time	Meal Plans	Serving Size	Carbs (grams)
_____	**Breakfast**		
	Protein		
	Fruit or grain		
	Beverage		
_____	**Protein Snack**		
_____	**Lunch**		
	Protein		
	Vegetable		
	Lettuce		
	Fruit		
	Beverage		
	Miscellaneous		
_____	**Protein Snack**		
_____	**Dinner**		
	Protein		
	Vegetable		
	Lettuce		
	Fruit		
	Beverage		
	Miscellaneous		
_____	**Protein Snack**		
		TOTAL	

Keto Reading _____
Weight _____
Vitamins   AM   Noon   PM
Water _____

Activities _____
_____
_____

Pedometer Steps _____

WEEKLY BODY MEASUREMENTS

Chest _____   Hips _____
Waist _____   Thighs _____
Abdomen _____

SUCCESS LEARNING TOOLS

Read pages # _____
Audio Tape _____
Video _____
CD-ROM _____
Bio-Card ™ _____
Affirmation _____
_____

Other _____
Plan to Overcome Today's Obstacles:
_____
_____
_____
_____

Notes: _____
_____
_____
_____
_____

CHOOSE ONE DAY EACH WEEK AS YOUR "PROTEIN DAY."

ANY QUESTIONS?

Q: *When shouldn't I exercise? When should I take it slow?*

A: Skip your regular exercise whenever you have a fever. (If your fever is caused by a viral infection, exercise can increase the risk of the virus causing inflammation of your heart muscle.) If you've been away from your ordinary routine for four days or more, it's a good idea to ease back into it gradually. After any injury or surgery, it's a good idea to consult with your health professional before returning to exercise.

Q: *Is it okay to skip a day if I just don't feel like exercising?*

A: Okay with whom?

DAY 16

IF YOU WANT TO CHANGE YOUR BODY, YOU HAVE TO CHANGE YOUR MIND

You can learn to tell your brain what to tell your body.

If you've ever lost weight and then regained it—as most of us have—the mental training techniques you'll be learning today may be just the "something" you need to get off the diet roller coaster once and for all.

What you think, how you feel, how you plan, and what you expect determines the decisions you make and how well you carry them out. By strengthening the connection between your body and your mind, you can enhance your success.

Here's how the nurses in our clinics explain the process:

1. *Your brain tells the rest of your body what to do.* It sends messages by way of nerve signals and chemicals released into the bloodstream. These messages influence your body's structure, functioning, and observable actions.

2. *Your brain knows what the rest of your body is doing.* The rest of your body sends messages back to the brain.

3. *You can tell your brain what to tell your body right now.* You can trigger short-term changes inside your body, and you can enact whatever actions you have decided to carry out.

4. *You can post instructions inside your brain to be used later.* Your brain is like a computer. It can be programmed to activate a certain function at a later time. You can let your brain know what messages to send to the rest of your body when you are under stress, paying attention to something else, or acting automatically, out of habit.

TELL ME MORE

Until recently, medical students were taught that the structure of the brain changed very little after childhood. Only within the past 15 years have scientists discovered that the physical connections among nerve cells in the brain evolve throughout our lives as we continue to have life experiences. These patterns determine what messages the brain sends to the body and the conditions under which those messages are sent. What's more, we now know that we can change and strengthen these patterns if we so choose.

It's exciting to be able to tap into the incredible power that exists within us. It's especially intriguing to know that power can be accessed quickly to help achieve a specific goal. I know this can happen because I've done it. During an especially demanding three-month period several years ago, I was called upon to make a major presentation at a national medical convention. I also wanted to participate in a business-related golf tournament, even though I hadn't picked up a golf club in nearly five years. These events both surfaced at a time when I was developing a long-range strategic plan for Lindora that had to be completed for a presentation.

I knew something had to give—but what? The questions were more obvious than the answers. Could I do it all? Could I do it all *well*? How would I deal with the emotional, physical, and intellectual challenges that awaited me? How could I most effectively rally my resources to achieve my goals?

Once I clarified the challenge, I was determined to find the answers. I sought out Herman M. Frankel, M.D., and Jean Staeheli of Portland Health Institute, Inc., in Portland, Oregon. I was familiar with their groundbreaking mental training work and extraordinary success with Olympic and other world-class athletes, classical musicians, corporate executives, patients facing major surgery, people with chronic illness, trial witnesses, and others confronting life crises or crossroads. I was curious whether I could effectively apply their techniques to achieve my business-related goals, as well as to my goal of quickly enhancing my golf game.

In working with Frankel and Staeheli, I learned that mental activity can change brain structure and function, and *intentional mental*

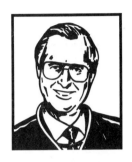

DR. STAMPER

"Train the brain and the body will follow! The mental training techniques described today are extremely powerful. When practiced consistently, they can help you enhance your performance in many areas of your life."

Lean *for* Life®
DAILY ACTION PLAN

Week _____ Day _____ Date _____

Time	Meal Plans	Serving Size	Carbs (grams)
	Breakfast		
	Protein		
	Fruit or grain		
	Beverage		
	Protein Snack		
	Lunch		
	Protein		
	Vegetable		
	Lettuce		
	Fruit		
	Beverage		
	Miscellaneous		
	Protein Snack		
	Dinner		
	Protein		
	Vegetable		
	Lettuce		
	Fruit		
	Beverage		
	Miscellaneous		
	Protein Snack		
		TOTAL	

Keto Reading _____
Weight _____
Vitamins   AM   Noon   PM
Water _____

Activities
_____
_____

Pedometer Steps _____

WEEKLY BODY MEASUREMENTS

Chest   Hips
Waist   Thighs
Abdomen

SUCCESS LEARNING TOOLS

Read pages # _____
Audio Tape _____
Video _____
CD-ROM _____
Bio-Card™ _____
Affirmation _____

_____
Other _____
Plan to Overcome Today's Obstacles:
_____
_____
_____
_____
_____

Notes:
_____
_____
_____
_____
_____

CHOOSE ONE DAY EACH WEEK AS YOUR "PROTEIN DAY."

activity can change brain structure and function as intended. In other words, we can change the physical structure of our brains through mental rehearsal just as we can through repeated physical rehearsal. When done properly, mental training is effective because, to a great extent, the effect on the brain is the same whether or not the practice we do is visible to others.

I found out that basketball players who *mentally* practice free throws can improve their performance at least as much as the player who actually spends the same amount of time practicing on the court. *The brain makes no distinction between physical practice and mental practice, so long as the mental training is done effectively.* This realization was important to me. I would need to prepare if I was going to participate in the golf tournament, yet I had little time to physically practice my game.

In the weeks that followed my initial work with Frankel and Staeheli, I discovered how to apply the mental training techniques that had supported countless Portland Health Institute clients to achieve optimal performance under stressful circumstances.

The effort paid off. My medical convention presentation exceeded my expectations. The golf tournament? Not only did I have a wonderful time, I played well enough to help my team win a first place trophy. The strategic planning was equally successful. In fact, the book you're holding is one of the results.

My experiences convinced me beyond any doubt just how powerful the connection between the brain and the body can be.

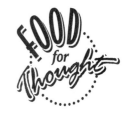

"If it were easy, everyone would do it."

— William Zinsser

Another Lean for Life Success Story

"The first time I did mental training, I felt a little self-conscious. I had a tough time staying focused. But then I reminded myself that if I had all the answers, I wouldn't be lugging around 75 extra pounds. I had nothing— and everything—to lose by giving it my best shot. I've achieved my goal and am using mental training techniques I learned on the program to train for my first marathon."

— *Joshua*

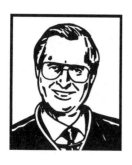

DR. STAMPER

"Is your ketostick
positive? Remember:
You're either in
ketosis or you're not!
If you're not, make
an immediate
adjustment to correct
the situation. See
page 29 for
a quick review."

techniques that work well for us, we want to share them with our patients to help them achieve greater results on the program. MENTORS Daily Mental Training became, and remains, an integral component of the Lean for Life program.

Our patients use a series of pre-recorded MENTORS Daily Mental Training tapes created especially for our program. Information on how to order the tapes series can be found on page 253. You can also make your own tape, using the script featured in today's "Your Turn."

Anyone can do mental training. At first, you may feel a little self-conscious. Be patient. You'll get better with practice. There's a reason that thousands of people, including athletes, musicians, business professionals, teachers, students, and, yes—dieters—are using this form of mental training. It works!

Now you can learn one more way to strengthen the connection between your brain and body and function more effectively than ever before.

During each Daily Mental Training session, you will be able to:

❑ Intentionally create a peaceful, receptive, undistracted state of mind;

❑ Experience yourself doing those things you've decided are important to you, achieving whatever personal goals you've set and feeling pleased at what you're doing;

❑ Complete the exercise by returning to your usual, alert state of mind, more comfortable and pleased with yourself than before.

MENTORS™ DAILY MENTAL TRAINING: HOW TO DO IT

Choose a quiet place where you can be undisturbed for 15 minutes. Since you will be achieving a more relaxed state of consciousness during this process than you are used to, *never do* MENTORS *Daily Mental Training while driving a car or operating any machinery or equipment*

Make yourself comfortable, either lying down or sitting, and close your eyes. If you become aware of any noises or distracting thoughts during your session, simply refocus your attention.

This narration is intended as a guide for creating your own tape. Some people read the instructions silently several times, then recreate them in their mind as they do the session. You might also ask a friend or family member to read them to you or to prepare a tape for you.

The following narrative is an abridged version of the MENTORS Daily Mental Training "Inner Mental Room" audiocassette. You may want to

The following narrative is an abridged version of the MENTORS Daily Mental Training "Inner Mental Room" audiocassette. You may want to use this narrative exactly as written for the first few sessions. With experience, you'll naturally find yourself elaborating in your own way and tailoring it to your needs.

It's helpful to decide what you want to be able to *do*, how you want to be able to *feel,* or how you want to be able to *be* before you begin the session. You can then experience yourself doing it successfully throughout the session. Examples could include: "In this session, I want to…

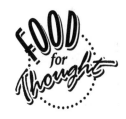

"Where the mind dwells, the body tends to follow."

—David Higdon

❑ experience myself at the beach, feeling good about my body."

❑ be calm and focused during my meeting this afternoon."

❑ be able to enjoy the party tomorrow night without letting food be the focus."

You want to experience—in as much sensory detail as you can—doing, feeling, or being whatever you have decided is important to you.

TAPE SCRIPT:

"When you are ready, you will be able to let your attention rest on your breathing. You can experience the air entering your body with each breath in, and you can experience the breath leaving your body every time you breathe out.

If you like, you can let yourself be aware of one part of your body at a time, letting yourself recognize a little bit of tightening, and the sensation of your own strength, as you breath in… then, as you breathe out, a letting go of whatever tightness you no longer need. You can feel a sensation of comfort and safety.

When you are ready, you can let yourself float down gradually… safe, strong, and co mfortable, to a spot from which you can enter your Inner Mental Room. You can let yourself be in your Inner Mental Room, where you know you are safe and secure. You can look around you, and see that you have everything you need. You can arrange your Inner Mental Room exactly as you choose, with whatever furnishings, equipment, and supplies you select.

When you are ready, you can let yourself become aware of a big screen in your Inner Mental Room. On this screen, you can let yourself see the place where you are doing what you are ready to be doing. You can be aware of the time of day, the presence of any people you choose, the details of your surroundings.

You can let yourself hear the sounds of this place … you can feel the gentle touch of the air on your face, and you can feel what's

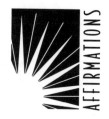

"I am enjoying taking
time for myself."

beneath you, comforting and reassuring. You can let yourself smell the aromas of this place, and even become more aware of the taste in your mouth. When you are ready, you can become aware of yourself, feeling safe, strong, and comfortable. You can let yourself look exactly as you are ready to look, and feel a sense of confidence and satisfaction as you let yourself do what you have decided is important to you...safe and strong and comfortable.

When you are ready, you can let yourself become aware again of being in your Inner Mental Room. You can let yourself return here any time you choose to do the mental training work that you have decided is important to you. Each time you let yourself be in your Inner Mental Room, you can feel a deep sense of confidence in your ability to work toward whatever goals you have chosen.

When you are ready, you'll be able to use your breathing in to help you raise your energy level. With each breathing in, you'll be able to become more fully awake and alert, relaxed, and refreshed. And then, when you're ready, you'll be able to breathe in and out two more big breaths, bend and straighten your elbows two times, and again become awake and alert, relaxed, refreshed... able to open your eyes and feel so good all over that you'll be able to feel just...like...smiling!"

THE RIGHT STUFF

Now that you've been exercising regularly for a couple of weeks, you may be thinking about investing in a good pair of walking shoes.

Good walking shoes provide cushioning and support, maximizing comfort and minimizing the risk of injury. Find an athletic shoe store with a knowledgeable sales staff. A good salesperson won't just hand you a box, but will work with you to find the right pair of shoes—one that fits your needs and price range.

ANY QUESTIONS?

Q: *Do Olympic and other world-class athletes really use the kind of mental training techniques I've just learned about?*

A: Absolutely. One of the most high-profile users of mental training techniques is Mike Powell, since 1990 the world's top-ranked long jumper.

Powell's "impossible dream" was to break the world long-jump record set in 1968 in the high, thin air of Mexico City. In early 1991, he began working with Herman M. Frankel, M.D. at Portland Health Institute. Many times each day over the course of seven months, Powell practiced the MENTORS Daily Mental Training techniques featured in this chapter. He mentally experienced himself jumping successfully in a variety of settings, weather conditions, and stressful situations. He practiced dealing with many different obstacles and distractions. He even mentally rehearsed his physical and emotional state during and after the setting of the new world record.

Powell's efforts paid off in a big way. At the 1991 World Championships in Tokyo, Powell jumped 29 feet, 4½ inches, shattering track and field's longest-standing record and establishing a new level of human accomplishment.

DAY
17

"WHY ARE YOU DOING THIS TO ME?"

You will learn how to deal successfully with those who try to sabotage your success.

S urprise!" David shouted from the kitchen as Sheila entered the house. "You'll never guess what we're having for dinner."
Sheila didn't need to guess. The aroma of pepperoni pizza was a dead giveaway, and Sheila was not pleased. It was the second time in two weeks that David "surprised" her with a tasty, high-fat, high-carbohydrate indulgence from their favorite Italian restaurant.

It just doesn't make sense," Sheila said with a shrug. "David tells me he's thrilled that I decided to lose weight. But as soon as I lose a few pounds, he starts undermining my success. I can't help but wonder 'What's going on here?'"

If you've ever tried losing weight before, chances are you understand Sheila's frustration. Perhaps it was your mother who insisted on making her famous homemade pork sausage lasagna. It may have been the workout buddy who told mutual friends how great you're doing but refused to compliment you face to face. Maybe it was your sister, who sent that two-pound box of gourmet chocolates for your birthday even though she knew you were determined to avoid fat and sugar.

You know they love and care about you... so why do they behave in ways that feel more like sabotage than support?

WHAT MOTIVATES DIET SABOTEURS?

By now it should come as no surprise that many people are threatened by change.

In some situations, the people around you may genuinely believe they want you to achieve your goal, yet fear that you—or their relationship with you—may somehow change if you succeed. They prefer the balance and order of your existing relationship—the way things are—over the unknown and the way things might be. This undermines their ability to support you. They become "diet saboteurs," often without realizing what they're doing.

It's also possible that your newfound self-control is making your diet saboteurs feel self-conscious, stirring concerns that if you look better, it will make them look worse. Maybe they're comfortable being the one with the nice body or pretty face while you're the one with the "great personality." Your progress may also be a reminder that they are no closer to their own goals than they were a year ago.

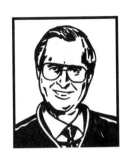

DR. STAMPER

"Asking for something greatly increases your odds of getting it."

It's important to understand that while diet saboteurs can be maddening, their behavior is seldom premeditated or intentionally cruel. When Sheila asked David, "Why are you doing this to me? Don't you want me to lose weight?" he was dumbfounded. "Of course I do!" he responded.

But Sheila found David's words inconsistent with his recent actions and she told him so. During one of their talks, David eventually acknowledged that perhaps he was feeling "a little threatened" by Sheila's determination to lose the 50 pounds she had gained since their wedding three years earlier.

"He told me it always bothered him when other men used to turn to look at me," Sheila says. "That rarely happened when I was heavier, which suited him just fine. Once we talked about how his inner conflicts were getting in the way of supporting me to achieve something I really wanted, we were able to work it through. Now he's reassured that he's the man for me and I feel better knowing he really has my best interest at heart. We've been walking together every night. What began as a conflict ended up being a real gift to our relationship."

There's an important lesson here. Open, honest communication can cut through the cobwebs of misunderstanding, unspoken feelings, and unresolved conflicts.

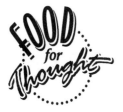

"The greatest

pleasure in life

is doing what

people say

you cannot do."

—Walter Bagehot

A FOUR-STEP STRATEGY FOR DEALING WITH SABOTEURS

The next time you believe someone is interfering with your weight loss, deal with it directly. Confrontation is rarely necessary, but candor is. This four-step approach will help:

1. *State the problem*. Be specific. Example: "I'm committed to my weight-loss program, but it's not always easy. When you offer me potato chips, it only makes it more difficult."

2. *Explain how you feel about the problem and why you need help with the resolution*. Example: "I'm frustrated. I know you care about me, but some of the things you've been doing lately are making it tough. You mean a lot to me and I know this is something we can work through."

3. *Detail what you want*. Don't assume the other person will instinctively know how to provide support. Example: "I'd like it if our time together didn't center on food so often. Instead of meeting for dinner next week, why don't we take in a movie or go for a walk at the park?"

4. *Describe the results you expect and the benefits of your success*. This is an opportunity to reaffirm your goal. Example: "I'm going to feel and look healthier, and I want you to know how much it means to me to know you're supporting me."

Is asking for support always easy? No. But as Sheila will tell you, it's definitely worth the effort.

Who are *your* diet saboteurs? Take a closer look at your relationship with each of the people who came to mind and ask yourself the following questions:

❏ What do you think motivates them to sabotage your weight-loss efforts?

❏ Are they usually supportive in other parts of your life?

❏ If so, what can they do—or stop doing—to be more supportive? If they are *never* supportive, what are you getting out of the relationship that motivates you to continue it?

Lean *for* Life®
DAILY ACTION PLAN

Week _____ Day _____ Date _____

Time	Meal Plans	Serving Size	Carbs (grams)
_____	**Breakfast**		
	Protein		
	Fruit or grain		
	Beverage		
_____	**Protein Snack**		
_____	**Lunch**		
	Protein		
	Vegetable		
	Lettuce		
	Fruit		
	Beverage		
	Miscellaneous		
_____	**Protein Snack**		
_____	**Dinner**		
	Protein		
	Vegetable		
	Lettuce		
	Fruit		
	Beverage		
	Miscellaneous		
_____	**Protein Snack**		
		TOTAL	

Keto Reading _____

Weight _____

Vitamins ____ AM ____ Noon ____ PM ____

Water _____

Activities _____
_____
_____
_____

Pedometer Steps _____

WEEKLY BODY MEASUREMENTS

Chest _____ Hips _____

Waist _____ Thighs _____

Abdomen _____

SUCCESS LEARNING TOOLS

Read pages # _____

Audio Tape _____

Video _____

CD-ROM _____

Bio-Card ™ _____

Affirmation _____

_____

Other _____

Plan to Overcome Today's Obstacles:
_____
_____
_____
_____
_____

Notes: _____
_____

CHOOSE ONE DAY EACH WEEK AS YOUR "PROTEIN DAY."

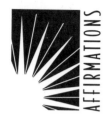

AFFIRMATIONS

"I am enjoying my new sense of well-being."

REFOCUSING ON YOUR VISION

Have you looked at your personal Vision Statement since you completed it two days ago? Take time today—and every day throughout your program—to review it until it feels like a part of you. It's also a good idea to revise and update your Vision Statement periodically. Many of the skills you're learning in this book, including affirmations, positive self-talk, and problem-solving strategies, will help support you in achieving your vision.

ANY QUESTIONS?

Q: *How many mental training sessions should I do each day? I'm very busy.*

A: One session a day can make a difference. Even greater benefits will result whenever you can squeeze in a second or third session. Keep track of your mental training work on your Daily Action Plan and observe the results. As long as you're making time for at least one session each day, you'll be in a position to decide how important it is for you to find time to do more.

Q: *I'm on the road nearly an hour every day. Why can't I do my MENTORS Mental Training while I'm driving?*

A: Unlike other mental training activities you'll be mastering in this program, your MENTORS Mental Training sessions will help you develop an ability to enter a peaceful state of mind, not unlike the state right before you fall asleep. The electrical activity of your brain will differ from that of your normal waking state. In this state, you are free to experience your mental activity and not pay attention to what's going on around you. To drive or operate any machinery could be dangerous to you and others.

YOUR MENTAL BLUEPRINT: WHO—AND HOW—ARE YOU SUPPOSED TO BE?

You can conquer the psychological causes of cravings by redefining your self-image and redrawing your "mental blueprint" of who you are and what you deserve.

For years, Dr. Stamper has believed that losing weight and keeping it off has at least as much to do with what we put in our *minds* as what we put in our *mouths*. That's because how we think and what we expect from—and for—ourselves directly impacts how we eat and how well we take care of our bodies.

As we grew up, we each developed our perspective as to how we—and our lives—were *supposed* to be. Our sense of right and wrong, good and bad, acceptable and unacceptable were influenced by our upbringing, experiences, and social conditioning. This belief system resulted in a "mental blueprint" of who we are and what we think we deserve.

Let's say that your blueprint of your physical self is of a thin, fit person. If so, you're much more likely to stay thin and fit because that's what your blueprint calls for. If you were to start gaining weight, you would be highly motivated to take the necessary steps to lose the weight, because being fat wouldn't match your blueprint of how you are supposed to be. It wouldn't be "you."

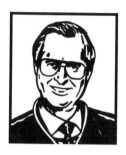

DR. STAMPER

"The most important

words you'll ever

hear are the ones you

tell yourself."

Likewise, if your mental blueprint is of an overweight person, you will be predisposed to do whatever it takes to remain overweight. As long as that blueprint is in place, you will fight to maintain it, *especially if you begin losing weight.* You will be inclined, without realizing it, to sabotage yourself by doing whatever it takes to ensure that your reality resembles your blueprint as closely as possible.

Your blueprint of how things are *supposed* to be influences how things actually *are.* As long as you leave the old blueprint in place, any weight loss or "remodeling" you accomplish isn't likely to last long. Why? Because when you lose weight, your reality will be out of synch with how you are "supposed" to be. Straying too far from your mental blueprint stirs inner conflict.

This reaction has nothing at all to do with being "stupid," "bad," or "stubborn." It has everything to do with being human. When our reality doesn't match our blueprint, we tend to change the reality until it does. By understanding this idea, we can recognize that the problem contains the seeds of the solution.

Let's say, for example, that right this minute you want to eat. You're experiencing cravings and can't identify any physical causes or environmental cues for your sudden urge to eat.

What would happen if you took this opportunity to look at your mental blueprint? Ask yourself the following questions:

❏ "What do I think I'm supposed to look like?"

❏ "What does my mental blueprint say I'm supposed to be doing in this situation?"

❏ "If my mental blueprint shows an overweight person, what might I do in this situation to achieve that blueprint?"

SO WHAT'S THE SOLUTION?

Once you explore these questions, the solution will become obvious—change the blueprint! Replace your "fat" blueprint with a more appropriate one.

You want to fill your mind with images of yourself being energetic, slender, and strong. You want to see yourself moving effortlessly. You want to look at others who have the kind of body you want and see yourself in the same way. You want to identify characters in movies and on television who resemble how you intend to look once you've lost your weight.

Lean *for* Life®
DAILY ACTION PLAN

Week _____   Day _____   Date _____

Time	Meal Plans	Serving Size	Carbs (grams)
_____	**Breakfast**		
	Protein		
	Fruit or grain		
	Beverage		
_____	**Protein Snack**		
_____	**Lunch**		
	Protein		
	Vegetable		
	Lettuce		
	Fruit		
	Beverage		
	Miscellaneous		
_____	**Protein Snack**		
_____	**Dinner**		
	Protein		
	Vegetable		
	Lettuce		
	Fruit		
	Beverage		
	Miscellaneous		
_____	**Protein Snack**		
		TOTAL	

Keto Reading _____

Weight _____

Vitamins   AM   Noon   PM

Water _____

Activities _____
_____
_____

Pedometer Steps _____

WEEKLY BODY MEASUREMENTS

Chest _____   Hips _____

Waist _____   Thighs _____

Abdomen _____

SUCCESS LEARNING TOOLS

Read pages # _____

Audio Tape _____

Video _____

CD-ROM _____

Bio-Card™ _____

Affirmation _____
_____
_____

Other _____

Plan to Overcome Today's Obstacles:
_____
_____
_____
_____
_____

Notes:
_____
_____
_____
_____

CHOOSE ONE DAY EACH WEEK AS YOUR "PROTEIN DAY."

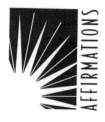

AFFIRMATIONS

"I am enjoying
turning my
obstacles into
opportunities."

There are more deliberate ways to establish and maintain the blueprint you want. You already have access to a variety of tools that can effectively put new blueprints, patterns, and expectations in place. You know about using BioModifiers to change what's going on inside. You can use powerful positive affirmations to shape your expectations and actions. You can use your mental training sessions to put new images in place.

In the days ahead, you'll learn more ways to change what's inside, so that when you get what you expect, it will be what you really want and you'll be ready to enjoy it.

JERRY SEINFELD CAN MAKE YOU FAT

Have you ever grabbed the cookies or potato chips as you tuned in your favorite television show, only to realize later than you almost ate the entire bag?

It's easy to do. When your attention is focused elsewhere, you can be unaware of what—and how much— you're eating. To avoid this trap, limit your eating to one area of your home, preferably your kitchen or dining room table. And when you eat, focus on your meal. Turn off the TV, put down the paper and enjoy the taste, texture, and aroma of the food.

OVERCOMING PLATEAUS

You can overcome temporary stalls and setbacks to achieve your weight-loss goal.

Don't be discouraged if at some point during "Phase 1: Weight Loss," you experience what's commonly known as a weight-loss "plateau." A plateau is nothing more than a short period of time, usually one to seven days, during which your body will temporarily resist losing weight. Even though you're following the program carefully, the same number on the scale stubbornly stares back at you.

As you can imagine, plateaus are maddening. After all, most of us believe that if we play by the rules, we'll win. It can be discouraging and demoralizing to do it "right" and not experience the expected payoff.

If you allow them to, plateaus can undermine your self-confidence. They can leave you questioning whether the program "works" and even lead you to overeat out of sheer frustration.

That's why it's so important to understand what plateaus are, why they occur, and how to move beyond them.

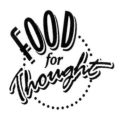

WHAT CAUSES PLATEAUS?

In some cases, plateaus are the result of water retention. If you're retaining water while losing fat, the scale won't necessarily reflect the fat loss. And since water weighs more than fat, it's even possible to lose fat while retaining water and have the scale actually reflect a weight gain.

Some people also experience a plateau whenever they return to a weight to which their body is accustomed. Let's say you started the program weighing 150 pounds and your goal is 125. If you've weighed 135 pounds for years, you may experience a plateau when your body returns to that weight. This kind of "body memory" is common. The body achieves a "comfort zone" that it strives to maintain. No one is certain exactly why this happens, but our experience over millions of treatment sessions tells us it does.

THE GOOD NEWS ABOUT PLATEAUS

All this talk about plateaus may sound pretty grim. But there is good news: *they're only temporary!* It's important to recognize plateaus for exactly what they are. Rather than thinking of them as defeats, derailments, or detours, realize that they're nothing more than temporary road blocks.

Remember:

❏ Plateaus are not permanent.

❏ They are not proof that you "can't lose weight."

❏ Above all, they are no excuse to lose your enthusiasm, momentum, or focus.

IT'S NOT A PLATEAU IF. . .

Now that you understand what a plateau is, it's equally important to recognize what a plateau is not. If you're *not* losing weight and you're *not* in ketosis, you are *not* experiencing a plateau. To convince yourself otherwise is to sabotage your success. *A true plateau occurs only when you are in ketosis and are temporarily not losing weight.*

When you are doing the program correctly, you *will* be in ketosis. Ketosis occurs whenever a person limits his or her carbohydrate intake to between 50 and 100 grams daily. If you're not in ketosis, you're burning carbohydrates—not fat—as your primary energy source.

Those carbohydrates are coming from somewhere. Be honest with yourself. Are you aware of everything you're eating? Read

Lean *for* Life®
DAILY ACTION PLAN

Week _____ Day _____ Date _____

Time	Meal Plans	Serving Size	Carbs (grams)
	Breakfast		
	Protein		
	Fruit or grain		
	Beverage		
	Protein Snack		
	Lunch		
	Protein		
	Vegetable		
	Lettuce		
	Fruit		
	Beverage		
	Miscellaneous		
	Protein Snack		
	Dinner		
	Protein		
	Vegetable		
	Lettuce		
	Fruit		
	Beverage		
	Miscellaneous		
	Protein Snack		
	TOTAL		

Keto Reading _____
Weight _____
Vitamins   AM _____   Noon _____   PM _____
Water _____

Activities _____
_____
_____

Pedometer Steps _____

WEEKLY BODY MEASUREMENTS
Chest _____   Hips _____
Waist _____   Thighs _____
Abdomen _____

SUCCESS LEARNING TOOLS
Read pages # _____
Audio Tape _____
Video _____
CD-ROM _____
Bio-Card™ _____
Affirmation _____
_____

Other _____
Plan to Overcome Today's Obstacles:
_____
_____
_____
_____

Notes: _____
_____
_____
_____
_____
_____

CHOOSE ONE DAY EACH WEEK AS YOUR "PROTEIN DAY."

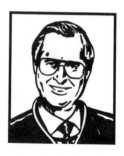

DR. STAMPER

"If you don't take

care of your body,

where are you

going to live?"

labels carefully to make sure you're not consuming hidden carbohydrates. Measure portions. Take special care in maintaining your Daily Action Plan. You may want to do one or two Protein Days until you're back in ketosis, then resume your Weight Loss menu.

If you *are* in ketosis and experiencing a plateau, you may wish to use the Plateau Menu below for *no more than three days* or until you "break" your plateau by losing 1½ pounds or more, whichever comes first.

THE BOTTOM LINE ON PLATEAUS

Stay focused on your goal and remember that plateaus are temporary. Your patience and persistence will pay off. While it's natural to want what you want when you want it, there are times when your body has a mind of its own. Choose to keep your goal in sight.

Continue
to have
protein snacks
while on a
plateau

THE LEAN FOR LIFE PLATEAU MENU

Breakfast
   1 egg or egg substitute (boiled, poached, or cooked
      with Pam in a nonstick pan)
   ½ grapefruit
   Choice of any calorie-free beverage

Lunch
   3½ ounces, white fish
   ½ cup, cooked spinach
   ½ grapefruit
   1 cup, lettuce
   Choice of any calorie-free beverage

Dinner
   3½ ounces, white fish
   ½ cup, cooked spinach
   ½ grapefruit
   1 cup, lettuce
   Choice of any calorie-free beverage

At Bedtime
   1 cup, hot lemon water (¼ lemon, boiled in water
      for three minutes)

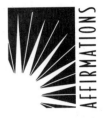

ANY QUESTIONS?

Q: I'm exercising every day and really starting to see and feel results. Exactly what effect does exercise have on my muscles?

A: Exercise changes the way your muscles *work*, the way they *feel*, and the way they *look*. It also improves:

❑ your strength (how much force you can exert; for example, how heavy a load you can carry)

❑ your stamina (how long or how many times you can carry it)

❑ your power (how far you can throw it)

❑ your agility (how gracefully you can move it)

❑ your flexibility (how far you can move it before your joints can't bend or straighten any more)

❑ your coordination (how well you can perform complex moves with it)

❑ your speed (how fast you can move with or without it)

❑ your ability to resist or recover from injury.

When you exercise regularly, your muscles—and you—become firmer and more appealing to look at and touch.

AFFIRMATIONS

"I am enjoying taking care of myself."

Another Lean for Life Success Story

"On every diet I ever tried, I hit a plateau, got discouraged, and gave up. Lean for Life is the only program that told me up front that plateaus were normal—and that they could be overcome. When I stayed stuck at 201 for four days, I was determined to break through it. And I did! I've been at my lean weight of 185 for nearly two years."

— Victor

THEN&NOW

YourTurn

It's been two weeks since we first looked at how environmental cues can trigger a desire to eat even when we're not hungry.

When was the last time you found yourself eating in response to an external cue such as a TV food commercial, a particular pastry shop, or the company of certain people?

_____

_____

What did you eat? _____

_____

How did you feel afterward? _____

_____

What could you have done instead? _____

_____

What did you learn? _____

_____

DAY 20

AFFIRMING THE POSITIVE

You can communicate with yourself in ways that affirm your ability to achieve your goals.

Have you ever had one of those truly perfect days when you felt capable, confident, and totally self-assured? You were ready for any challenge that came your way and felt thoroughly equipped to accomplish whatever you set your mind to. Those nagging inner voices—the ones that sometimes insist "I can't do this" or "I'm not good enough"—were nowhere to be heard.

You can have more of those days by using a simple but effective technique called affirmations. In just a few minutes every day, you can neutralize the effects of negative thinking on your mind and body, replacing them with a soothing, encouraging, optimistic way of thinking and feeling that will make your life more positive and successful.

Affirmations are positive, personal statements that you create, write down, and repeat to yourself to affirm, in your mind, that you're capable of accomplishing your goal.

ACCENTUATE THE POSITIVE

Effective affirmations highlight your *positive behavior* by stating what you are doing rather than not doing. Example: "I am eating

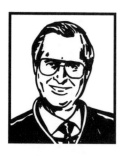

DR. STAMPER

"Negative thoughts
are like pebbles. If
you carry one or
two around, you
may not notice.
But when you
accumulate enough
of them, they really
weigh you down."

healthy foods that nourish my body" rather than "I am not eating junk food anymore." They also highlight your *positive feelings* by describing what you want rather than what you don't want. Example: "I am becoming healthy, strong, and lean" rather than "I don't want to be fat anymore." What's more, they also underscore your *positive commitment* by focusing on firm statements ("I am succeeding at becoming Lean for Life") rather than tentative or predictive statements ("I hope to become Lean for Life").

An easy way to remind yourself of the positive foundation of affirmations is to visualize yourself moving actively and happily toward what you want instead of running away from what you don't want.

At first, the notion of being able to enhance your self-confidence by making positive statements about yourself may sound like little more than New-Age psychobabble. But while "the power of positive thinking" may be a cliche, the fact is positive thinking *can* be powerful! Research suggests that affirmations can have a significant psychological impact on our emotions and health by neutralizing the unconscious negative beliefs and feelings that undermine so many people's success.

WHEN TO DO AFFIRMATIONS

Many of our patients recite an affirmation before they get out of bed in the morning and in the evening as they prepare to fall asleep. That way, the affirmation is the first and last message they hear each day. These are the times when you're most likely to be in a relaxed, receptive state of mind. In order for the affirmation to become a routine part of your thinking, it's necessary to experience it in a deeper, more "whole body" kind of way rather than merely on a "thinking" level.

An affirmation that comes from your heart will always be appropriate for you, even when you're asserting something that doesn't feel quite real yet. If you deliver the message to yourself often enough, it will begin to feel real. And that's the point. You make a choice as to how you want to be and then help yourself become that person.

Lean *for* Life®
DAILY ACTION PLAN

Week _____ Day _____ Date _____

Time	Meal Plans	Serving Size	Carbs (grams)
_____	**Breakfast**		
	Protein		
	Fruit or grain		
	Beverage		
_____	**Protein Snack**		
_____	**Lunch**		
	Protein		
	Vegetable		
	Lettuce		
	Fruit		
	Beverage		
	Miscellaneous		
_____	**Protein Snack**		
_____	**Dinner**		
	Protein		
	Vegetable		
	Lettuce		
	Fruit		
	Beverage		
	Miscellaneous		
_____	**Protein Snack**		
		TOTAL	

Keto Reading _____
Weight _____
Vitamins   AM _____   Noon _____   PM _____
Water _____

Activities _____
_____
_____
_____

Pedometer Steps _____

WEEKLY BODY MEASUREMENTS
Chest _____   Hips _____
Waist _____   Thighs _____
Abdomen _____

SUCCESS LEARNING TOOLS
Read pages # _____
Audio Tape _____
Video _____
CD-ROM _____
Bio-Card™ _____
Affirmation _____
_____
Other _____
Plan to Overcome Today's Obstacles:
_____
_____
_____
_____
_____
Notes:
_____
_____
_____
_____

CHOOSE ONE DAY EACH WEEK AS YOUR "PROTEIN DAY."

FOOD for Thought

"You never lose until you stop trying."

—Mike Ditka

Your Turn

As you prepare to create your affirmations, remember that they are always personal "I" statements. That's because they're about you and no one else. Also be sure that your affirmations are stated in the present tense. Say "I am..." rather than "I will..." and you will come from a position of having already achieved your stated desire.

Now that you have an understanding of affirmations and how you can benefit from using them, it's your turn to come up with some you can use. These sample affirmations may spark some ideas:

- ❑ "I have everything I need to be healthy."
- ❑ "The food I'm eating makes me healthy and lean."
- ❑ "I feel wonderful when I exercise."
- ❑ "I am filled with energy."
- ❑ "I am a problem solver."
- ❑ "I can handle whatever challenges life gives me."
- ❑ "I am proud of myself for being a patient, kind person."
- ❑ "I am enjoying becoming Lean for Life."
- ❑ "I am having fun being active."
- ❑ "I am becoming healthy, strong, and lean."
- ❑ "I am smiling."
- ❑ "I am sticking with my program."

Write three affirmations on a sheet of paper. Revise them until they feel right to you. Do they highlight your positive feelings? Do they encourage positive behavior? Do they affirm your positive commitment? Are they "I am" statements?

Once you're satisfied with your affirmations, write them here:

Affirmations

1. _____

2. _____

3. _____

Starting today, choose one of your affirmations and repeat it throughout the day. The more often you repeat your affirmation, the more it will become a part of you and the way you see the world.

VISUALIZATIONS:
WHAT YOU GET IS WHAT YOU SEE

You can learn to diffuse negative self-talk
by visualizing your success.

Ask anyone who knows William and they'll tell you he's one of the nicest people you'd ever want to meet. And he is—to everyone but himself.

While he's understanding and easy-going with his wife, children, friends, and employees, the 42-year-old landscaper never realized how hard he was on himself. Then one morning, his Lindora nurse suggested he write down every negative thought he had and every negative comment he made about himself for the rest of the day.

By noon, William's list already included: 9:26AM: "I really blew it!" ... 10:15AM: "At the rate I'm going I'm never going to lose these last 10 pounds!" ... 10:38AM: "Gee, I'm about as sharp as a marble!" ... 11:20AM: "What a klutz!" ... 11:55AM: "I'm absolutely terrible at remembering names!"

The exercise was quite an eye-opener. William suddenly realized how unforgiving and judgmental he was with himself—totally different from the way he was with loved ones, friends, or even casual acquaintances.

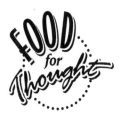

William's not unique. Many of us surrender undeserved power to our negative inner voices. What's more, while we're quick to label our "failures" as being "bad" or "stupid," we're rarely as willing to give ourselves credit when things go well.

In fact, some of us react to our successes as harshly as we do our setbacks, dismissing our accomplishments ("I was lucky"), minimizing our achievements ("It was no big deal"), and even predicting future failure ("I never do things right twice in a row—I'll probably mess up tomorrow!"). When was the last time you said to yourself, "I did that exactly the way I wanted to and it was terrific?"

While this kind of negative self-talk may not sound damaging, it takes a toll. What we say to ourselves tends to be a predictor of what will actually happen. The steady drip of negative messages can eventually wash away our self-esteem and confidence in our ability to function effectively in the world.

Recognizing how you talk to yourself is important because *what you say to yourself in any particular setting has a profound effect on how you are likely to perform in that setting in the future*. When you tell yourself something often enough, you begin to believe it. You begin to "see" it in your mind.

The scenes you play in your head change your brain structure. These scenes are examples of BioModifiers, those things we do on purpose to help ourselves get what we want by changing what's happening inside our brains. As the scene that you visualize and store in your brain becomes more and more familiar, it will begin to play itself out that way more predictably and more often, because you will start functioning in the ways that have become more familiar to you.

That's why many world-class athletes and classical musicians include mental rehearsal of their routines and emotions prior to a competition or performance. They also mentally replay the details of their successes after every event, mentally revising imperfect moments so that what gets stored in their memories is a successful execution of the task rather than an unsuccessful one.

You can learn how to use the same kind of powerful, brief visualizations for specific purposes. Whether you're preparing to exercise, about to enter a restaurant, or contemplating a decision, you can pause briefly to visualize the scene exactly as you would like to see it play out, complete with sound, sensation, aroma, taste, and emotion.

A brief visualization differs from a Mentors Daily Mental Training session or other mental training in that it's shorter and can take place when you're fully alert. It's totally focused on one scene and is typically done immediately before you begin or resume an activity in your

Lean *for* Life®
DAILY ACTION PLAN

Week _____   Day _____   Date _____

Time	Meal Plans	Serving Size	Carbs (grams)
_____	**Breakfast**		
	Protein		
	Fruit or grain		
	Beverage		
_____	**Protein Snack**		
_____	**Lunch**		
	Protein		
	Vegetable		
	Lettuce		
	Fruit		
	Beverage		
	Miscellaneous		
_____	**Protein Snack**		
_____	**Dinner**		
	Protein		
	Vegetable		
	Lettuce		
	Fruit		
	Beverage		
	Miscellaneous		
_____	**Protein Snack**		
		TOTAL	

Keto Reading _____
Weight _____
Vitamins   AM _____   Noon _____   PM _____
Water _____

Activities _____
_____
_____

Pedometer Steps _____

WEEKLY BODY MEASUREMENTS
Chest _____   Hips _____
Waist _____   Thighs _____
Abdomen _____

SUCCESS LEARNING TOOLS
Read pages # _____
Audio Tape _____
Video _____
CD-ROM _____
Bio-Card ™ _____
Affirmation _____

Other _____
Plan to Overcome Today's Obstacles:
_____
_____
_____
_____

Notes:
_____
_____
_____
_____

CHOOSE ONE DAY EACH WEEK AS YOUR "PROTEIN DAY."

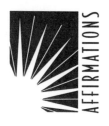

AFFIRMATIONS

"I feel terrific when I eat nutritious, healthy food."

everyday life. A brief visualization may be used as a positive response to negative self-talk because it replaces a negative pattern with an emotionally positive one. Similarly, brief visualizations can be used immediately after you've experienced a disappointment or failure, or immediately before starting a challenging activity.

Brief visualizations can be done at any time. They don't require time alone, closing your eyes, or entering an alterative state of consciousness. They simply require that you remind yourself of your power to create the positive mental state that leads to success.

Go ahead. Do it. See what happens.

THE HIDDEN PAYOFFS OF BEING FAT

If you had asked Colleen a year ago to tell you about the benefits of being fat, she would have denied there were any.

But today—after losing 109 pounds and gaining a greater sense of awareness—the 32-year-old entertainment attorney knows better.

"Not only did I drop the weight, but I dropped the defenses that helped make me fat in the first place," she explains. "There were benefits I wasn't even aware of until I had to give them up. My weight was a convenient excuse for anything that wasn't working in my life. If I lost a case, for example, I would tell myself it was because the jury didn't like fat women. One day it dawned on me—my fat was taking a toll on my self-respect as well as on my body."

Several months into her program, Colleen also came face-to-face with a truth she had long denied: for 10 years she had been using her fat to insulate herself from men.

"I was never comfortable with all of the attention I got from boys in high school," she explains. "The more weight I put on, the less of a problem it was. Without my realizing it, this was my way of protecting myself. At that point in my life, it never occurred to me that I could be a thin, attractive woman and not be hassled or harrassed by men."

What have been *your* hidden payoffs for being overweight? One of the main themes of this book is awareness. By clearly identifying benefits you derived from being overweight, you will take an important first step toward ensuring that you don't lapse into self-defeating patterns of behavior.

6

WEIGHT LOSS
WEEK 4

THE POWER OF PRACTICE

You will learn how consistency, repetition, and practice can help you maintain the results you've achieved.

It's a joke as old as the Empire State Building: A tourist approaches a Manhattan street musician near Central Park and says, "Excuse me, sir, how do I get to Carnegie Hall?"

As the musician's bow dances across the strings of his violin, he grins and replies, "Practice, my friend, practice!"

As tired as it is, this joke illustrates a relevant point: to maintain any degree of success, you must *keep* doing what you've been doing to achieve the results you're currently enjoying.

It all boils down to "use it or lose it," a cliche that also happens to be an absolute truth. As renowned pianist Artur Rubenstein once observed, "If I miss one day, I can tell; if I miss two days, the audience can tell."

Like Rubenstein, you need to keep up with your daily regimen, too. By doing gentle exercise, you'll maintain the increased mitochondria and increased insulin receptors you've built up in your muscle cells.

It's equally important that you continue your mental training. It results in specific changes in the circuits of connections among brain cells and in brain chemistry that will work to your advantage.

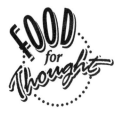

And just like physical training, in which many athletes cross-train by blending strength training, flexibility training, and speed training into an overall regimen, mental training is also "cross-trainable."

Since you have a variety of mental training tools available to choose from—including positive affirmations, MENTOR Daily Mental Training sessions, your personal Vision Statement, Motivator cards, and brief visualization techniques—you have plenty of opportunities to do different kinds of mental training without the process ever becoming boring or tedious.

So keep it up! You've invested too much to get where you are to run the risk of returning to where you were!

ACTIVITY BY THE NUMBERS

Ever wonder how many calories you were burning while standing, swimming, or shoveling snow?
With this chart, you'll know.

Calories Burned During 15 Minutes of Activity

Activity	125 lbs.	175 lbs.	250 lbs.
Sleeping	15	21	30
Standing	18	24	36
Walking (4 mph)	78	108	153
Climbing stairs	219	303	432
Cycling (13 mph)	133	186	267
Washing windows	52	72	103
Shoveling snow	97	133	195
Light office work	37	51	75
Carpentry	48	66	96
Chopping wood	90	126	181
Basketball	87	123	175
Dancing (vigorous)	72	99	141
Golfing	49	72	102
Racquetball	112	156	216
Water skiing	90	132	195
Swimming (crawl)	60	84	120
Volleyball	64	97	141

Lean *for* Life®
DAILY ACTION PLAN

Week _____   Day _____   Date _____

Time	Meal Plans	Serving Size	Carbs (grams)
_____	**Breakfast**		
	Protein		
	Fruit or grain		
	Beverage		
_____	**Protein Snack**		
_____	**Lunch**		
	Protein		
	Vegetable		
	Lettuce		
	Fruit		
	Beverage		
	Miscellaneous		
_____	**Protein Snack**		
_____	**Dinner**		
	Protein		
	Vegetable		
	Lettuce		
	Fruit		
	Beverage		
	Miscellaneous		
_____	**Protein Snack**		
		TOTAL	

Keto Reading _____
Weight _____
Vitamins   AM   Noon   PM
Water _____

Activities _____
_____
_____

Pedometer Steps _____

WEEKLY BODY MEASUREMENTS
Chest _____   Hips _____
Waist _____   Thighs _____
Abdomen _____

SUCCESS LEARNING TOOLS
Read pages # _____
Audio Tape _____
Video _____
CD-ROM _____
Bio-Card™ _____
Affirmation _____

Other _____
Plan to Overcome Today's Obstacles:
_____
_____
_____
_____

Notes:
_____
_____
_____
_____

CHOOSE ONE DAY EACH WEEK AS YOUR "PROTEIN DAY."

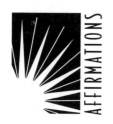

AFFIRMATIONS

"I enjoy my exercise."

EXERCISING YOUR OPTIONS: MAKING FITNESS FUN

After you've done anything for a few weeks, your initial enthusiasm can begin to fade. But your exercise routine doesn't have to be routine at all. Here are three tips to help you stay moving and motivated:

1. *Set short-term goals.* Whatever your ultimate fitness goal happens to be, you're more likely to achieve it if you divide it into smaller, less imposing intermediate goals. Rather than committing to an hour of exercise, five times a week for the next year, focus instead on the present and the immediate future. What are you realistically willing and able to commit to during the next two weeks? Thirty minutes? Forty? Three times a week or four? Write your commitment down and then do it. Keep a written record of your exercise accomplishments in a notebook. During this two-week period, assess your exercise and activities and renew your commitment to the process.

2. *Schedule exercise into your day.* Whenever you make a business, social, or medical appointment, you probably write it down in your calendar. You consider it a commitment and you don't want to forget. As you begin your fourth week of the program, think of your exercise time as an appointment with yourself. Schedule it in just as you would a dental appointment or dinner with a friend—and then keep the date!

3. *Remember that when it comes to exercise, anything is better than nothing.* No matter how stressed, busy, or exhausted you are, it's important that you exercise—even if only for a brief time. Make a deal with yourself that on your scheduled workout days, you'll squeeze in at least a light, 20-minute workout, no matter what.

   Be resourceful. This might mean taking a brisk walk through the airport as you wait for a flight. It could mean stretching in your office while returning phone calls or using your coffee break as an exercise break. Instead of strolling down to the cafeteria, go outdoors for a brisk 10-minute walk. Take the stairs instead of the elevator. Rather than circling for a close parking space, park your car in the first space you see and walk to your destination.

   Any movement is better then none, so do what you can. The more demanding your day, the more valuable this break will be.

A HEALTHY INVESTMENT

*You will learn to identify the "ingredients"
you consider important for a healthy life.*

If you were asked to share your "recipe" for a healthy life, which essential "ingredients" would top your list?

As you begin your last week of "Phase 1: Weight Loss," it's a question well worth asking—and answering. Before you read any further, take a few minutes and write down what you consider to be the basic components of a healthy, balanced life:

_____

_____

_____

_____

_____

_____

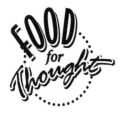

Our years of clinical experience have taught us that certain "ingredients" are essential. How does your list compare to this one, which was developed with our friends at Portland Health Institute?

H   Higher purpose
E   Eating healthy food
A   Activity that is gentle and regular
L   Laughter and play
T   Time alone
H   Human contact

Higher purpose. People who feel more fulfilled are those who live with a sense of purpose and passion, commit to ideas and ideals greater than themselves, and give of themselves without expectation of personal gain. What do *you* believe in? What stirs your passions? How often do you lend your time and talent to causes and concerns that matter to you?

Eating healthy food. Even though you're currently in the weight-loss phase of the program, your ultimate goal is to develop a healthy way of eating that will serve you well for the rest of your life. As you know, the emphasis is on plenty of fruits and vegetables, protein for energy and muscle building, moderate carbohydrates, and little fat. Once you've lost all the weight you want to lose, you'll see the benefits of moderation and common sense in maintaining your weight loss.

Activity that is gentle and regular. Activity is vital in the life of anyone who truly wants to live well. We're only beginning to understand how our miraculous bodies manage to function so beautifully. But one thing we do know is that the human body was designed for movement, and all of our mental and physical systems

THE BUDDY SYSTEM

You might be surprised to discover how willing one of your friends, neighbors, or co-workers would be to join you in your exercise routine. The support and structure that the "buddy system" offers will keep both of you motivated. It's easy to break promises to yourself. But when you know someone is waiting for you at the gym or at the beginning of your walking trail, you're much more likely to show up. And when you do, you both benefit!

Lean *for* Life®
DAILY ACTION PLAN

Week _____ Day _____ Date _____

Time	Meal Plans	Serving Size	Carbs (grams)
	Breakfast		
	Protein		
	Fruit or grain		
	Beverage		
	Protein Snack		
	Lunch		
	Protein		
	Vegetable		
	Lettuce		
	Fruit		
	Beverage		
	Miscellaneous		
	Protein Snack		
	Dinner		
	Protein		
	Vegetable		
	Lettuce		
	Fruit		
	Beverage		
	Miscellaneous		
	Protein Snack		
		TOTAL	

Keto Reading _____
Weight _____
Vitamins   AM   Noon   PM
Water _____

Activities _____
_____
_____
_____

Pedometer Steps _____

WEEKLY BODY MEASUREMENTS

Chest _____   Hips _____
Waist _____   Thighs _____
Abdomen _____

SUCCESS LEARNING TOOLS

Read pages # _____
Audio Tape _____
Video _____
CD-ROM _____
Bio-Card™ _____
Affirmation _____

Other _____
Plan to Overcome Today's Obstacles: _____
_____
_____
_____
_____

Notes: _____
_____
_____
_____
_____
_____

CHOOSE ONE DAY EACH WEEK AS YOUR "PROTEIN DAY."

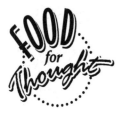

depend on keeping our bodies in good working order. Is your body getting enough movement?

Laughter and play. When we laugh, our bodies work better, our relationships work better, and our work works better. Henry Wheeler Shaw once commented that "laughter is the sensation of feeling good all over and showing it principally in one place." Not only does a good laugh feel good, it *does* good. Laughter is one of the ultimate BioModifiers. It helps nurture the soul. A sense of humor and an ability to play can be true lifesavers even in the darkest times. We need to remind ourselves to balance the serious with the playful. When was the last time you told a joke? Flew a kite? Walked in the rain? Surprised a friend or loved one with a relaxing day trip?

Time alone. "If one sets aside time for a business appointment or shopping expedition," Anne Morrow Lindbergh once observed, "that time is accepted as inviolable. But if one says, 'I cannot come because that is my hour to be alone,' one is considered rude, egotistical, or strange. What commentary on our civilization."

As the pace of contemporary life seems to ever-accelerate, it's easy to forget what Lindbergh clearly realized—that time alone is time well spent. Solitude allows the soul time to reflect upon itself. There is an emotional clarity and inner calm that can occur only when we're alone, reflecting and thinking without interruption. Thomas Edison suggested that "the best thinking has been done in solitude; the worst has been done in turmoil." When we hop off life's treadmill for some "alone time" every now and then, we recharge the spirit and renew our sense of wonder and joy in life. When is the last time you spent a quiet afternoon alone, with no radio, reading, or rules? Do you do it as often as you'd like? Why not?

Human contact. The connection to others through words and touch is life itself. We are made for it. And when we don't get enough of it, we tend to become depressed and sick more often. Fortunately, we all possess the power to initiate and maintain contact with the world around us. How good are you at staying connected?

Are your "HEALTH" needs currently being met in ways you find satisfying? In which of these six categories do you feel most fulfilled? Which could use a little more attention?

Take time to treat yourself well. "HEALTH" is an investment in yourself. And like any good investment, it will pay off.

ANY QUESTIONS?

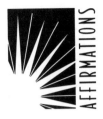

AFFIRMATIONS

Q: *I'm doing my gentle exercise every day but I don't like it. Any suggestions?*

A: There's a big difference between activity not being your favorite thing and being something you truly dread. Try defining what it is about exercise that you don't like.

Be specific. Is it having to shower afterward? Maybe you could walk first in the morning before you shower and get ready for work. Is it lonely? What not invite a friend to come along? Is it the weather? You could always drive to a nearby shopping mall and walk there. What specific solutions can you think of for overcoming your discomfort?

It's possible that no solutions will come to mind or will feel right. Under these circumstances, you can remind yourself that exercise is valuable, even on those days when you don't feel like doing it. This gives you the freedom to address the question, "Is it OK for me to do something I don't like if I have reason to think it will help me achieve my goals?"

Review your Motivator cards whenever you feel yourself losing momentum and motivation. This will help you shift your focus to why you're doing the program and how much you enjoy the benefits.

"I appreciate my body and feel good about the changes I see."

DAY 24

SUCCESS STRATEGIES: MEETING "REAL LIFE" CHALLENGES

You will discover simple but effective strategies for successfully managing the temptations that life presents.

No matter how motivated and determined you are to stick with your plan to lose weight, there are going to be times when "real life" presents situations that heighten temptation and lower your resistance.

But that doesn't suggest you have to become a victim of circumstance. By anticipating everyday challenges and approaching them with a Plan of Action, you can sidestep the predictable pitfalls that derail many dieters.

Today and tomorrow, we'll take a look at a number of potentially difficult "real life" situations—everything from grocery shopping to ordering in restaurants to eating on the run—and offer practical strategies to help you stay focused on results. First, let's discuss one of the biggest traps—and how to avoid falling into it.

MARKETING 101

A trip to your neighborhood grocery store can be a true test of will. They're strategically designed to stimulate impulse buying, and their marketing tactics work. There are, however, ways you can level the playing field the next time you go shopping:

Review your Motivator card. Before you go food shopping, review your reasons for becoming Lean for Life. This will help you stay focused and motivated.

Never shop when you're hungry. Always eat a meal or a protein snack first.

Avoid shopping when you're stressed and/or tired. The more frazzled you are, the more likely you'll be to buy impulsively. If you're used to shopping on your way home from work, try going either early in the morning when you're rested or later at night after you've had dinner and time to relax.

Steer clear of your "danger zones." For some, that may be the store bakery. For others, it's the aisle stocked with nuts, potato chips, and other salty snacks. You know your danger zones better than anyone. By avoiding them, you'll reduce the temptation to buy "a little bag" of this or "just one box" of that.

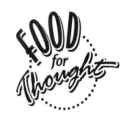

"If you have the will to win, you have achieved half your success. If you don't, you have achieved half your failure."
—David Ambrose

"MR. MITO" SAYS:

"Ever heard of the Toothbrush Tush Push or the Towel Toner? They're "bonus" exercises you can do in your bathroom while getting ready in the morning. Like most exercises, they're more fun when you do them to music.

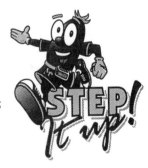

❑ *Toothbrush Tush Push: The music's playing and there's toothpaste on the brush. Stand tall with your feet apart and your toes turned out. As you brush, bend and then straighten your knees to the music. Who would have ever guessed that good oral hygiene could also result in a firmer rear end?*

❑ *Towel Toner: Stand with your feet apart. Grab a towel with both hands, then raise your arms above your head and pull the towel taught. Bend from side to side, at least 12 times each. Make it fun by getting with the beat of the music.*

Sure, they sound silly—but extra exercises like these can eventually result in bonus benefits you can see!"

Serving sizes are now more consistent across product lines, stated in both household and metric measures, and reflect the amounts people actually eat.

The list of nutrients covers those most important to the health of today's consumers, most of whom need to worry about getting much of certain items (fat, for example), rather than too few minerals, as in the past.

The label now tells the number of calories per gram of fat, carbohydrates, and protein.

Nutrition Facts

Serving Size ½ cup (114g)
Servings Per Container: 4

Amount Per Serving

Calories 90	Calories from Fat 30

	% Daily Value*
Total Fat 3g	5%
Saturated Fat 0g	0%
Cholesterol 0 mg	0%
Sodium 300mg	13%
Total Carbohydrate 13g	4%
Dietary Fiber 3g	12%
Sugars 3g	
Protein 3g	

Vitamin A 80% • Vitamin C 60% • Calcium 4% • Iron 4%

*Percent Daily Values are based on a 2,000 calorie diet. Your Daily Values may be higher or lower depending on your calorie needs:

Nutrient		2,000 Calories	2,500 Calories
Total Fat	Less than	65g	80g
Sat Fat	Less than	20g	25g
Cholesterol	Less than	300mg	300mg
Sodium	Less than	2,400mg	2,400mg
Total Carbohydrate		300g	375g
Fiber		25g	30g

Calories per gram:
Fat 9 • Carbohydrates 4 • Protein 4

Calories from fat are now shown on the label to help consumers meet dietary guidelines that recommend people get no more than 30 percent of their calories from fat.

%Daily Value shows how a food fits into the overall daily diet.

Daily values are also something new. Some are maximums, as with fat (65 grams or less); others are minimums, as with carbohydrates (300 grams or above). The daily values on the label are based on a daily diet of 2,000 and 2,500 calories. Individuals should adjust the values to fit their own calorie intake.

Learn to read food labels. Labeling reforms mandated by the Food and Drug Administration have made food labels much more "user friendly" but they can still be confusing. Take a look at the food label above. What would you say is the percentage of fat?

If you answered five percent, you'd be making a very common error. Take a closer look at the "Calories from Fat." Each serving contains 90 calories, and 30 of those calories are from fat. That means this food is *33% fat!* The "Total Fat" percentage of five percent simply indicates that a single serving of this food provides five percent of the daily value, *based on a 2,000 calorie diet.*

Always shop from a list. If it's not on your list, don't buy it. This simple strategy will save you time, money, and unwanted calories.

Lean for Life®
DAILY ACTION PLAN

Week _____ Day _____ Date _____

Time	Meal Plans	Serving Size	Carbs (grams)
_____	**Breakfast**		
	Protein		
	Fruit or grain		
	Beverage		
_____	**Snack**		
_____	**Lunch**		
	Protein		
	Vegetable		
	Lettuce		
	Fruit		
	Beverage		
	Miscellaneous		
_____	**Snack**		
_____	**Dinner**		
	Protein		
	Vegetable		
	Lettuce		
	Fruit		
	Beverage		
	Miscellaneous		
_____	**Snack**		
		TOTAL	

Keto Reading _____
Weight _____
Vitamins   AM _____   Noon _____   PM _____
Water _____

Activities _____
_____
_____

Pedometer Steps _____

WEEKLY BODY MEASUREMENTS
Chest _____ Hips _____
Waist _____ Thighs _____
Abdomen _____

SUCCESS LEARNING TOOLS
Read pages # _____
Audio Tape _____
Video _____
CD-ROM _____
Bio-Card ™ _____
Affirmation _____
_____
_____

Other _____
Plan to Overcome Today's Obstacles:
_____
_____
_____
_____
_____

Notes:
_____
_____
_____
_____
_____
_____

CHOOSE ONE DAY EACH WEEK AS YOUR "PROTEIN DAY."

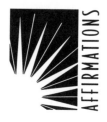

AFFIRMATIONS

"I am in control of

what I eat."

Shop less and buy more. The more often you visit the market, the more likely you are to buy food you don't need.

Buy fresh. When buying fruits and vegetables, remember that fresh is better than frozen, and frozen is better than canned.

Beware of misleading buzzwords. Food manufacturers are well aware that the American consumer is more health conscious today than ever before. It's no coincidence that so many food products are now being marketed as "Lite", "Low-Fat," and "Reduced Calorie." These products often deliver exactly what they promise and represent tasty alternatives to their higher-fat counterparts. But in some cases, the so-called "healthy" alternatives are as loaded with fat and sugar as the original products they pretend to improve upon.

Know what you're buying. Compare labels. "Lite" as opposed to what? "Lower in calories" than what? "Reduced" from what? Avoid becoming a victim of shrewd food marketing by shopping smart!

Tomorrow, we'll look at a number of other "real life" situations— and how you can successfully face the challenges they present.

PUT YOUR MONEY WHERE YOUR MOUTH IS

A Michigan State University study found that people who bet $40 they could stick with their workout program for six months had a whopping 97% success rate. Only 20% of those who didn't make the bet followed through on their program. Challenge your workout buddy. The first one to slack off pays up!

TAKING THE OFFENSIVE: OVERCOMING OTHER "REAL LIFE" TEMPTATIONS

You'll learn how to neutralize five everyday danger zones and stay focused on your goal.

While that trip to the grocery store can be a tormenting test of self-control and willpower, it's certainly not the only "real life" situation that can jeopardize your success. Today let's focus on five other situations in which temptation looms large. By using a combination of the 20 success strategies offered here, you can neutralize temptation's impact and stay focused on your weight-loss goal.

HAVE IT YOUR WAY

Whoever said eating in restaurants has to be an ordeal just because you're on a weight-loss program? In fact, you can learn how to turn dining out into an enjoyable, stress-free event. Here are some of the success strategies our patients find most helpful:

Choose restaurants carefully. If you're not sure whether a restaurant serves chicken or fish, call ahead and ask. Avoid "all you can eat" buffets and restaurants known for huge portions. It'll be much easier for you to stick with your program if you're not sitting

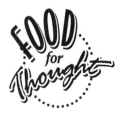

across from a friend who's devouring the "Mother Lode" mega-platter of nachos.

Speak up. If a friend or business associate suggests meeting at a restaurant where you think you might have a tough time ordering food you can eat, don't hesitate to suggest alternatives: "I'd love to meet you for lunch, but instead of pizza, let's try that new seafood restaurant down the street." You'll discover that most people are fairly flexible, especially if you tell them why you're making your suggestions.

Avoid temptation by avoiding the menu. That's right—don't even read it. Instead, tell the server exactly what you would like. Surprisingly, this is just as easy to do in inexpensive coffee shops and chain restaurants as it is in elegant five-star establishments. The restaurant business is extremely competitive, and most restaurants are more than willing to satisfy health-conscious customers by preparing food to order.

Be specific when ordering. If you want your entree broiled, baked, or grilled, be sure to say so. Ordering what you want might sound something like this: "I'd like a skinless chicken breast, grilled or broiled, some steamed vegetables without butter, and a small green salad with vinegar on the side." If it's not prepared properly, have them try again.

Steer clear of the dessert tray. If you're sure that a restaurant typically presents a dessert tray, tell your server before you finish your entree that you won't be having dessert. If you'd like fresh fruit, ask what is available. Again, it's a matter of planning ahead and exercising control.

Always keep an "emergency supply" of protein snacks in your briefcase, car, and office. If you find yourself in a dining situation where it's truly impossible to order well, order light and satisfy your hunger later with a protein snack.

NOW YOU'RE COOKING

You can create delicious meals for yourself and your family while you're becoming Lean for Life. In fact, you'll probably find that food tastes better, because you'll be preparing it in healthier ways. Make a point to:

Prepare only one evening meal. Period. If you cook one meal for your family and another for yourself, you'll likely end up feeling

Lean for Life®
DAILY ACTION PLAN

Week _____   Day _____   Date _____

Time	Meal Plans	Serving Size	Carbs (grams)
_____	**Breakfast**		
	Protein		
	Fruit or grain		
	Beverage		
_____	**Protein Snack**		
_____	**Lunch**		
	Protein		
	Vegetable		
	Lettuce		
	Fruit		
	Beverage		
	Miscellaneous		
_____	**Protein Snack**		
_____	**Dinner**		
	Protein		
	Vegetable		
	Lettuce		
	Fruit		
	Beverage		
	Miscellaneous		
_____	**Protein Snack**		
		TOTAL	

Keto Reading _____

Weight _____

Vitamins   AM   Noon   PM

Water _____

Activities _____
_____
_____

Pedometer Steps _____

WEEKLY BODY MEASUREMENTS

Chest _____   Hips _____

Waist _____   Thighs _____

Abdomen _____

SUCCESS LEARNING TOOLS

Read pages # _____

Audio Tape _____

Video _____

CD-ROM _____

Bio-Card ™ _____

Affirmation _____

_____

Other _____

Plan to Overcome Today's Obstacles:
_____
_____
_____
_____
_____

Notes:
_____
_____
_____
_____

CHOOSE ONE DAY EACH WEEK AS YOUR "PROTEIN DAY."

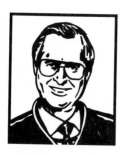

DR. STAMPER

"You are responsible.
You are in control.
You possess the
power to stay focused
on your goal and
achieve it."

deprived. Instead, make healthy, tasty meals that are on your program and can also be enjoyed by the entire family. Not only will you reduce your time in the kitchen, you'll also be including your family in a healthier way of eating.

Obesity tends to run in families—not only because of genetics, but because bad eating habits are often learned early in life. By encouraging your children to eat in more healthy ways, you can help them avoid many of the food-related challenges you find yourself facing today.

Delegate food-related duties. If you have children, have them help at mealtime. Younger children can set and clear the table. Older kids can help you prepare a salad.

Don't turn meals into a power struggle. Even the most health-conscious kids are not always going to want to eat what you're eating on the program. If they're old enough, let them prepare their own dinners once a week. Perhaps you can plan dinner out once a week so that everyone in the family can order what he or she wants.

Stick with the choices and portion sizes designated on your program. Just because some family members eat larger portions or have additional foods doesn't mean you have to. Don't let anyone else's appetite affect your success!

THE MORNING RUSH

A healthy breakfast is a great way to start the day, yet it's the meal that dieters are most likely to skip. No matter how busy you are, you can enjoy breakfast and still get to work on time:

Make time for it. Build breakfast into your morning—even if it means getting up 10 minutes earlier.

Plan ahead. Boil a dozen eggs at one time so you have plenty to last through the week. A few minutes before you walk out the door, drop a slice of bread in the toaster or take a piece of fruit and a container of nonfat yogurt out of the refrigerator, and pour yourself a cup of coffee. As you're heading to work, you can enjoy an easy-to-make breakfast that's much less expensive and better for you than the fast-food alternatives.

UNDER THE WEATHER?

Flu, colds, viruses, and other illnesses can take a real toll on your body. This is especially true whenever you're eating less food than normal. Since your body perceives any illness as a threat, it conserves energy (calories) and water in an effort to help you recuperate.

This basic biological fact can temporarily stall your weight-loss efforts. Don't get discouraged or distracted. Make getting well and feeling better a priority and continue on your program unless otherwise directed by your physician. As you begin feeling better, you'll overcome any temporary weight plateaus that you've experienced while recuperating.

Whenever you're not feeling well, be sure to:

Call or visit your doctor. Discuss your symptoms.

Carefully read labels on all over-the-counter medications. Choose pressed cold tablets such as Dristan or Comtrex. Many liquid medications and throat lozenges contain sugar and/or alcohol, both of which tend to stimulate appetite. They're loaded with extra calories, too.

Continue taking vitamins. Your daily supply (two vitamins, three times a day) contains 600 mg of Vitamin C, 10 times the U.S. recommended daily allowance.

Drink plenty of water and herbal teas. Make a point to stay hydrated even if you're not thirsty.

Don't skip meals. No matter how dull your appetite may be, it's essential that you get enough to eat—especially when you're not feeling well.

EATING ON THE JOB

It's happened to all of us. You're at work and you don't have time to get away for lunch. Those vending machines in the break room or cafeteria may seem like a quick fix—and they are. The problem, of course, is that a *quick* fix isn't always a *healthy solution*. But with a little advance planning, eating at work can be every bit as easy—and delicious—as eating at home:

Take your lunch. What better way to plan ahead—and guarantee that what you want will be available—than to make your own? If your workplace doesn't have a refrigerator you can use, carry your food in a small cooler. If you have access to a microwave, take prepared lunch entrees in plastic containers.

Don't skip your three daily protein snacks. Make a habit of taking your mid-morning and mid-afternoon snacks with you every morning. Keep a diet soda and a couple of protein snacks handy.

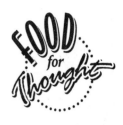

"Love yourself first and everything else will fall into line. You really have to love yourself to get anything done in this world."

—Lucille Ball

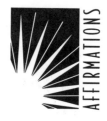

AFFIRMATIONS

Make healthy choices when ordering fast food. If a quick trip to a nearby fast-food restaurant is your only option, be cautious and think ahead. When you're hungry, it's easy to order impulsively and then regret it an hour later. Most fast-food places serve salads, and many offer char-broiled or grilled chicken. You can always order the grilled chicken sandwich and skip the bun.

No matter *where* you eat, the choice to eat well is always yours.

ANY QUESTIONS?

Q: *Does it matter what time of day I walk?*

A: What matters more than *when* you walk is *that* you walk. There is no one "right" time. The benefits you enjoy can vary depending on the time of day. Consider the "four S's" when deciding what's best for you:

❏ *Schedule*. When does your walk best fit into your schedule? When are you most likely to do it and enjoy it? When you plan an evening walk, do you usually do it or do you sometimes talk yourself out of it? If so, you'd probably be better off walking in the morning.

❏ *Safety*. Do you feel safe walking your favorite routes at the times that are best for you? Is there another place or a different time in which you'd be safer?

❏ *Sun exposure*. Schedule your walks with sun exposure and temperature in mind. Some people love the solar power that comes with the heat of the day. Others burn easily and find that too much sun saps their energy. Do whatever works for you—just be sure to protect your skin with sunscreen.

❏ *Side benefits*. Do you prefer the energizing benefits of an early-morning walk or the relaxing opportunity to unwind that results from walking at the end of the day? Many people find that a late-morning walk helps curb their appetite, while others value the "second wind" they get from walking mid-afternoon. Decide which "side benefits" are most important—and treat yourself to at least one dose a day.

GO WITH THE "FLOW"

You will learn about one of the rewards of engaging in activities such as exercise with commitment and concentration.

Imagine an experience so joyous and exhilarating that you would pursue it regardless of the obstacles, costs, or risks. While engaged in this adventure, feelings of self-doubt or self-consciousness would be nonexistent. You would be oblivious to time, and your concentration would be so total that you wouldn't worry or think about anything else.

Sound like a ticket you'd buy? An adventure you'd empty your savings account for? A dream you'd pursue? What if I told you that you could achieve this experience through physical activity? That's right. Physical activity. If you've been exercising regularly, you may have already experienced this remarkable state of mind that athletes and other achievers refer to as "flow."

Flow was first identified by University of Chicago psychologist Mihaly Csikszentmihalyi. In his book *Flow: The Psychology of Optimal Experience* (Harper & Row, 1990), Csikszentmihalyi describes this internal state as "so enjoyable that people will do it even at great cost, for the sheer joy of doing it," one in which people "are so involved in an activity that nothing else seems to matter."

Lean for Life®
DAILY ACTION PLAN

Week _____   Day _____   Date _____

Time	Meal Plans	Serving Size	Carbs (grams)
	Breakfast		
	Protein		
	Fruit or grain		
	Beverage		
	Protein Snack		
	Lunch		
	Protein		
	Vegetable		
	Lettuce		
	Fruit		
	Beverage		
	Miscellaneous		
	Protein Snack		
	Dinner		
	Protein		
	Vegetable		
	Lettuce		
	Fruit		
	Beverage		
	Miscellaneous		
	Protein Snack		
		TOTAL	

Keto Reading _____

Weight _____

Vitamins   AM   Noon   PM

Water _____

Activities _____
_____
_____

Pedometer Steps _____

WEEKLY BODY MEASUREMENTS

Chest _____   Hips _____

Waist _____   Thighs _____

Abdomen _____

SUCCESS LEARNING TOOLS

Read pages # _____

Audio Tape _____

Video _____

CD-ROM _____

Bio-Card™ _____

Affirmation _____

Other _____

Plan to Overcome Today's Obstacles:
_____
_____
_____
_____
_____

Notes: _____
_____
_____
_____
_____

CHOOSE ONE DAY EACH WEEK AS YOUR "PROTEIN DAY."

This state of mind has been studied in artists, factory workers, musicians, athletes, surgeons, homemakers, Buddhist monks, even a Japanese Hell's Angels motorcycle gang. Regardless of age, gender, ethnicity, cultural background, or type of activity, Csikszentmihalyi and his colleagues found the same pattern in people who are fully engaged in what they are doing—"a state of complete involvement and satisfaction."

Flow experiences rarely result from passive activities such as watching television. They are much more likely to occur when people do something that stretches their capacities, something that requires the full concentration of their abilities.

In a flow state, there's a perfect balance between the level of the challenge and your level of skill. The immediate consequence is that you are fully engaged in the activity. You're unburdened by any awareness of time, external distractions, the quality of your performance, and even yourself.

Flow is the experience that prompts people to think, "This is as good as it gets!" Your problems vanish and fresh solutions surface. You experience a liberating sense of harmony and safety that frees you to function more fully than before.

If you haven't felt it yet, stay active and interested. Before long, you're bound to experience the rush that results when you "go with the flow."

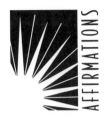

AFFIRMATIONS

"I appreciate my body and feel good about the changes I see."

IT SURE WORKED FOR THEM!

Albert Einstein, Charles Dickens, and Frank Lloyd Wright each knew the value of exercising their bodies as well as their minds. They were all inveterate walkers, often seen strolling through their neighborhoods during breaks from their respective work in physics, literature, and architecture.

While no one knows how often Webster went walking, you've got to love his definition of exercise: "the act of bringing into play or realizing in action; to use." After all, that's exactly what exercise is—*using* your body and realizing results through action!

Regular walks certainly seemed to work for these creative geniuses. Are you giving them a chance to work for you?

DAY 27

PREPARING FOR "PHASE 2: METABOLIC ADJUSTMENT"

You will learn more about the next phase of the program: how it works and how you'll benefit from doing it successfully.

Over the past month you've faced—and met—many challenges. You've had the opportunity to use new skills in overcoming obstacles. You've learned to be successful at losing weight. You're looking and feeling healthier than you did just four weeks ago. You're now ready to be successful at the greatest challenge of all—preparing to *maintain* the weight loss you've achieved.

Whether you're close to your goal or still have a way to go, you'll begin "Phase 2: Metabolic Adjustment" in just a couple of days. During this vital 14-day phase of the program, you will begin eating more food, making additions according to a specific schedule. You'll also continue maintaining your Daily Action Plan, exercising daily, and using the mental training techniques you find most helpful.

During Metabolic Adjustment, *the goal isn't to lose weight, but to gradually eat more without gaining weight.*

THE BENEFITS OF "PHASE 2: METABOLIC ADJUSTMENT"

During Phase 2, your body will:

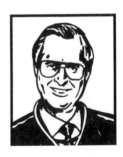

DR. STAMPER

"What your mind

can conceive, your

body can achieve."

❑ adjust to the fact that it has recently lost a significant amount of body fat, so that it will not start working desperately to replace it as soon as you begin to eat more calories.

❑ adjust your body chemistry back to a state in which you're not in ketosis and you are able to eat more carbohydrates again.

❑ physiologically begin the process of adjusting your setpoint to your new, lower weight so you can enjoy eating enough so you're not hungry but not so much that you'll regain weight.

❑ raise your metabolic rate so that you're burning more calories and are able to eat more food without gaining weight.

❑ restore the normal physiological pattern of using carbohydrate as well as fat for fuel.

Phase 2 is a time to take stock and take pride in what you've accomplished. It's also a time to stay focused.

Even though it's straightforward and easy to follow, "Phase 2: Metabolic Adjustment" is the part of the program in which people are most likely to make mistakes and interrupt their success.

Once you've completed this two-week process, you'll have a decision to make. You can either begin a second weight-loss series (of up to four weeks) or, if you've achieved your goal weight, you'll advance to the third and last phase of the program: Lifetime Maintenance.

MINI GOALS = MAJOR CHANGES

What will you accomplish *today*? For the next week, focus on one element of the program and challenge yourself to achieve a specific "mini-goal" every day, such as:

❑ logging 3,000 more steps on your pedometer.
❑ drinking 10 glasses of water.
❑ repeating an affirmation six times.

You'll soon find that you've effected a major change in how you feel and look. Remind yourself of your "mini-goal" several times during the day, and be sure to follow through. The sense of accomplishment you'll feel when you achieve it will keep you motivated.

Lean *for* Life®
DAILY ACTION PLAN

Week _____ Day _____ Date _____

Time	Meal Plans	Serving Size	Carbs (grams)
_____	**Breakfast**		
	Protein		
	Fruit or grain		
	Beverage		
_____	**Protein Snack**		
_____	**Lunch**		
	Protein		
	Vegetable		
	Lettuce		
	Fruit		
	Beverage		
	Miscellaneous		
_____	**Protein Snack**		
_____	**Dinner**		
	Protein		
	Vegetable		
	Lettuce		
	Fruit		
	Beverage		
	Miscellaneous		
_____	**Protein Snack**		
		TOTAL	

Keto Reading _____
Weight _____
Vitamins   AM   Noon   PM
Water _____

Activities _____
_____
_____

Pedometer Steps _____

WEEKLY BODY MEASUREMENTS

Chest _____   Hips _____
Waist _____   Thighs _____
Abdomen _____

SUCCESS LEARNING TOOLS

Read pages # _____
Audio Tape _____
Video _____
CD-ROM _____
Bio-Card ™ _____
Affirmation _____
_____
_____

Other _____
Plan to Overcome Today's Obstacles:
_____
_____
_____
_____
_____

Notes:
_____
_____
_____
_____
_____

CHOOSE ONE DAY EACH WEEK AS YOUR "PROTEIN DAY."

ANY QUESTIONS?

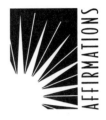

AFFIRMATIONS

Q: I find that walking really perks me up when I'm feeling depressed. It also calms me down when I'm feeling anxious. How does my body know which way to react to the same activity?

A: Getting "perked up" and "calmed down" may sound like movement in opposite directions, but think of them as moving toward the center, where mind and body are in balance. Walking and other gentle exercise can also:

❑ raise or lower your energy level, depending on whether you were feeling sluggish or overexcited when you started.

❑ help you become more alert or help you get ready for sleep, depending on whether you're just waking up or ending a long, full day.

Q: Why is it that I often find it easier to open up and have a meaningful discussion with someone when we're walking than when we're sitting across a table from one another?

A: Many people find that when they're physically active and moving in a continuous, easy rhythm, it's easier for them to think more clearly and communicate more openly. In this state, resistance is lowered and feelings of self-consciouness seem to diminish. If you're someone who derives these added benefits from walking, enjoy and make good use of it!

"I have confidence that I will succeed. "

DAY

28

THE PAST IS A PRESENT AS YOU PROCEED TO THE FUTURE

You'll focus on discoveries you've made and declare your intentions for applying them as you move into the next phase of the program.

Congratulations! Today you will complete the weight-loss phase of your Lean for Life program. You now stand at the gateway of "Phase 2: Metabolic Adjustment," ready to begin a 14-day period in which you'll learn how to gradually begin eating more food without regaining the weight you've just lost.

During the past four weeks, you've learned how to take care of yourself in new ways. You've acquired valuable new tools and discovered new approaches, strategies, and ideas for losing weight and improving your health. Every day of "Phase 1: Weight Loss" has been designed to empower you, to help you increase your awareness and knowledge, and to support you in taking greater responsibility for your body and your life.

Over the past four weeks you've undertaken a challenging personal journey. In the process, you've charted new territory; some days were undoubtedly more stimulating or stressful than others. But like the pieces of a puzzle, they ultimately fit together to create a finished product.

As you pause before beginning the next phase of your trip, it's time to take stock, to decide which tools and strategies you've found most useful in developing and maintaining your focus and commitment over the past four weeks. In other words, what newfound knowledge and awareness will be most valuable as you advance to "Phase 2: Metabolic Adjustment" and then on to "Phase 3: Lifetime Maintenance?"

We know from clinical experience that the people who continue to integrate the concepts of the program into their lives are the ones most likely to succeed at maintaining their weight loss. That's why today is devoted to looking back—and to focusing on how you can continue benefitting from your recent discoveries as you as move ahead.

SOLIDIFYING YOUR SUCCESS

The following exercise is one most people find fun and easy to do.

There are no right or wrong answers. What matters most is that you answer the questions thoughtfully. You may want to read each question, think about it for a few minutes, review the book briefly to refresh your memory, and consider all the ideas that come to mind. Then open your eyes and write down your answer.

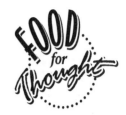

"There is no upper limit to what individuals are capable of doing with their minds... There is no obstacle that cannot be overcome if they persist and believe."

— E. F. Wells

1. **The most important thing I want to remember about** *my eating* **and weight loss is:**

   _____

   _____

   I can apply this in my life in the following ways:

   _____

   _____

2. **The most important thing I want to remember about** *my exercise* **and weight loss is:**

   _____

   _____

   I can apply this in my life in the following ways:

   _____

   _____

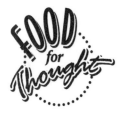

"The important thing is not where you were or where you are, but where you want to get."

—Dave Mahoney

3. **The most important thing I want to remember about** *my mental attitude* **and weight loss is:**

_____

_____

I can apply this in my life in the following ways:

_____

_____

4. **The most important thing I want to remember about** *my emotional health* **and weight loss is:**

_____

_____

I can apply this in my life in the following ways:

_____

_____

5. **The most important thing I can do to** *take care of myself* **as I move into the last two phases of the program is:**

_____

_____

I can apply this in my life in the following ways:

_____

_____

As you prepare to advance to the second phase of the program, let yourself reflect on the rewards you're enjoying as a result of your efforts. What changes do you most notice in your body? How do you look and feel today, compared to four weeks ago? Have the changes you're making in your body affected how you feel about yourself and how you relate to others?

Whatever benefits you're enjoying are enhanced by the fact you've earned them yourself. The progress you've made is a direct result of *your* actions, your willingness to set a goal and make it happen. In the process, you've demonstrated remarkable commitment and determination. You've invested energy, enthusiasm, and effort in the program and in yourself—and it's paying off. This will continue as long as *you* continue.

The first phase of this program has helped many thousands of people achieve their goal of becoming Lean for Life. The second and third phases of the program have helped them succeed in *staying* Lean for Life.

Let them do the same for you!

"MR. MITO" SAYS:

"How many steps have you logged on your pedometer today? Did you know the July 1996 report from the Office of the Surgeon General cautions that a "lack of physical activity is detrimental to your health"?

It's true. And guess what it recommends? A minimum of 30 minutes a day of moderate—i.e., gentle—exercise. So step to it!"

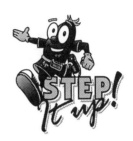

MEASURING UP

It's that time again! Measure your chest, waist, lower abdomen, hips, and upper thigh, and jot down the numbers below. How do they compare to the measurements you took back on Prep Day 2?

Chest _____   Hips _____

Waist _____   Thigh (upper) _____

Lower Abdomen_____

Lean for Life®
DAILY ACTION PLAN

Week _____   Day _____   Date _____

Time	Meal Plans	Serving Size	Carbs (grams)
_____	**Breakfast**		
	Protein		
	Fruit or grain		
	Beverage		
_____	**Protein Snack**		
_____	**Lunch**		
	Protein		
	Vegetable		
	Lettuce		
	Fruit		
	Beverage		
	Miscellaneous		
_____	**Protein Snack**		
_____	**Dinner**		
	Protein		
	Vegetable		
	Lettuce		
	Fruit		
	Beverage		
	Miscellaneous		
_____	**Protein Snack**		
		TOTAL	

Keto Reading _____
Weight _____
Vitamins   AM _____ Noon _____ PM _____
Water _____

Activities _____
_____
_____
_____

Pedometer Steps _____

WEEKLY BODY MEASUREMENTS
Chest _____   Hips _____
Waist _____   Thighs _____
Abdomen _____

SUCCESS LEARNING TOOLS
Read pages # _____
Audio Tape _____
Video _____
CD-ROM _____
Bio-Card™ _____
Affirmation _____

Other _____
Plan to Overcome Today's Obstacles:
_____
_____
_____
_____

Notes: _____
_____
_____

CHOOSE ONE DAY EACH WEEK AS YOUR "PROTEIN DAY."

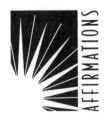

AFFIRMATIONS

"I am enjoying the
results of my efforts
and energy!"

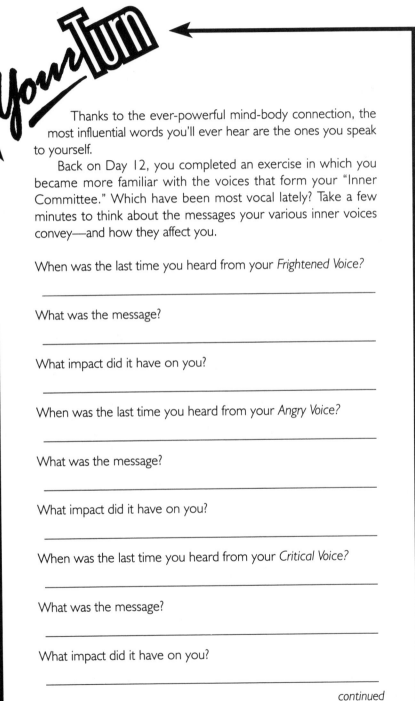

Thanks to the ever-powerful mind-body connection, the most influential words you'll ever hear are the ones you speak to yourself.

Back on Day 12, you completed an exercise in which you became more familiar with the voices that form your "Inner Committee." Which have been most vocal lately? Take a few minutes to think about the messages your various inner voices convey—and how they affect you.

When was the last time you heard from your *Frightened Voice?*

_____

What was the message?

_____

What impact did it have on you?

_____

When was the last time you heard from your *Angry Voice?*

_____

What was the message?

_____

What impact did it have on you?

_____

When was the last time you heard from your *Critical Voice?*

_____

What was the message?

_____

What impact did it have on you?

_____

continued

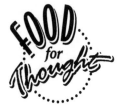

"The world is
for those who
make their dreams
come true."
— Harold Gray

When was the last time you heard from your *Joyful Voice?*

_____

What was the message?

_____

What impact did it have on you?

_____

When was the last time you heard from your *Curious Voice?*

_____

What was the message?

_____

What impact did it have on you?

_____

When was the last time you heard from your *Loving Voice?*

_____

What was the message?

_____

What impact did it have on you?

_____

When was the last time you heard from your *Confident Voice?*

_____

What was the message?

_____

What impact did it have on you?

_____

Remember: Speak nicely to yourself. Your brain hears you!

7

"PHASE 2: METABOLIC ADJUSTMENT"

You will be able to eat more food without gaining weight.

Anyone who has ever dieted knows that *losing* weight is only the first step. The challenge is keeping it off—and that's exactly what the second and third phases of the Lean for Life program are designed to help you accomplish.

After *every* four-week Weight Loss series you choose to do, you will move on to the second phase of the program: Metabolic Adjustment. During this 14-day phase, your goal will be to increase your body's metabolism, the rate at which you burn calories, by gradually increasing the amount of food you eat—without experiencing any weight gain.

Why, you may be wondering, is adjusting your metabolism so important? Whenever your body is forced to work on a reduced number of calories, as it's been doing during your weight-loss phase, it eventually adapts and trains itself to live on whatever calories it's getting—*without* losing weight. This built-in survival mechanism is called "metabolic adaptation." It's your body's way of protecting you against starvation. While metabolic adaptation can be a real lifesaver if you're stranded without food in the middle of nowhere, it can be a source of enormous frustration when you're eager to continue losing weight.

"Phase 2: Metabolic Adjustment" is a vital part of the program. It's also one of the most easily misunderstood. Many people—especially those who haven't yet achieved their Lean for Life goal—resist doing this phase of the program. And it's easy to understand why. After all, if you're still losing weight and you want to lose more, you want to keep doing what's working for you. It's easy to rationalize that taking a break from weight loss and adding new foods will only delay your progress.

In fact, the opposite is true. If you fail to complete this important second phase, you may soon find it difficult, if not impossible, to lose more weight. You may manage to lose a few "bonus pounds," but you'll lose them much more slowly. And before you know it, you're likely to regain those pounds—and more—whenever you begin eating more food.

If you *have* achieved your weight-loss goal, you may find yourself resisting the Metabolic Adjustment phase for different reasons. If you've lost all the weight you wanted to lose, it's easy to think that you've crossed the finish line, that you've succeeded. And you have—at least partially. But what you haven't done yet is taken the steps necessary to *maintain* your weight loss.

When you fail to adjust your metabolism, you set yourself up for a frustrating fall. That's because once you begin adding foods that are not part of Phase 2—or begin eating greater quantities of food—you will tend to gain weight rapidly because your body hasn't had a chance to adjust to the intake of extra "fuel." What it can't burn it stores as fat for future use. Even if you substitute foods that contain the same number of calories, you run the risk of decreasing your muscle mass and increasing your fat percentage. As a result, you may look and feel larger, even though your weight hasn't changed.

It's important for you to understand that the purpose of Metabolic Adjustment is *not* to lose weight, but to readjust your body's ability to metabolize an increasing number of calories. Since weight loss is not the goal of Phase 2, you will not be in ketosis during this part of your program. You will, however, continue doing one "Protein Day" during each week of Phase 2.

Metabolic Adjustment is an easy-to-follow process. The instructions for each of the three levels are very specific. Each level builds upon the one before it. Your menu choices during Phase 2 are identical to those in Phase 1.

As the chart on page 207 illustrates, the only difference between the Metabolic Adjustment phase and how you've been eating during Phase 1 is

METABOLIC ADJUSTMENT

LEVEL 1 (Days 1-3)	LEVEL 2 (Days 4-7)	LEVEL 3 (Days 8-14)
BREAKFAST		
2 Proteins	2 Proteins	2 Proteins
1½ Fruit or grain	1½ Fruit or grain	1½ Fruit or grain
1 Beverage	1 Beverage	1 Beverage
LUNCH		
1½ Proteins	2 Proteins	2 Proteins
1 Vegetable	1 Vegetable	1 Vegetable
Lettuce (unlimited)	Lettuce (unlimited)	Lettuce (unlimited)
1 Fruit	1 Fruit	1 Fruit
2 Misc.	2 Misc.	1 Grain
1 Beverage	1 Beverage	2 Misc.
		1 Beverage
DINNER		
1½ Proteins	2 Proteins	2 Proteins
1 Vegetable	1 Vegetable	1 Vegetable
Lettuce (unlimited)	Lettuce (unlimited)	Lettuce (unlimited)
1 Fruit	1 Fruit	1 Fruit
2 Misc.	2 Misc.	1 Grain
1 Beverage	1 Beverage	2 Misc.
		1 Beverage

that *some of your portion sizes are increased. The only addition of a new food during Metabolic Adjustment occurs on Day 8, when you'll begin adding a grain serving at both lunch and dinner.*

Your menu will continue to emphasize lean protein choices. Protein with each meal is essential to avoid triggering a carbohydrate/insulin

Another Lean for Life Success Story

"All my life people have called me stubborn. But I've always denied it because I am, of course, incredibly stubborn. I never realized exactly how bullheaded I could be until I lost, regained, lost, regained, and lost the same 20 pounds in less than two years! How did I do it? Skip Metabolic Adjustment and you'll find out for yourself.

"Every time I achieved my weight-loss goal, I figured I was home free. Even after I regained and lost the weight a second time, I convinced myself I could do it my way, that the second and third phases of the program were only for other people. I, of course, was 'special.'

"One day I was feeling very frustrated and made some comment to the effect that the program didn't work. Eva, my Lindora nurse, wasn't buying it. She pointed out that Phase 1 of the program had worked for me not once but three times, and that Phase 2 and Phase 3 hadn't 'worked' because I hadn't done them.

"As stubborn as I sometimes am, even I had to admit that Eva had a point. My problem wasn't with the program. It was my resistance to following directions, following through, and committing 100%. I realized I'd cheated myself out of a lot of benefits of the program, among them lasting results.

"Eva encouraged me to think of the second phase of the program as a step toward achieving 'metabolic fitness.' I continued exercising regularly and followed the three levels. Once I fully committed to doing it, I found I was able to tolerate more calories without gaining weight. I was also more satisfied with my meals and less tempted to snack.

"It's been nearly two years since I finished Metabolic Adjustment. During that time, I've maintained my 20-pound weight loss. Do I feel better physically? You bet. But what feels just as terrific is finally breaking free from a pattern that was leading to nothing but frustration."

—Fran

response, which can make you hungry and increase your likelihood of bingeing.

You will begin with Level 1, increasing quantities at breakfast, lunch, and dinner as indicated on your Daily Action Plan sheets included in this chapter. When you've increased food quantities as indicated on Level 1 and have maintained your weight within 1½ pounds (based on your weight when you began Metabolic Adjustment,) you'll move on to Level 2, repeating the same process before continuing to Level 3. Once you have gradually made these food changes over 14 days—and maintained your weight within 1½ pounds—you will have completed "Phase 2: Metabolic Adjustment."

Any time you experience a weight gain of 1½ pounds or more, substitute Lean for Life protein products or another protein choice for your dinner *that evening* and the extra weight should be gone the next day. You may need to do this for more than one day if you seriously overate. Do not move on to the next level of food addition until your weight is back within the 1½ pound range.

What makes 1½ pounds the "magic number"? First, your body weight can fluctuate that much for any number of reasons, so becoming concerned over a weight gain of a half-pound or even a pound can be much ado about nothing. The 1½-pound marker also establishes a clear guideline that will help you keep a minor fluctuation from becoming a major weight gain. No one gains 20, 30, or 50 pounds overnight. It sneaks up on you, a pound or two at a time. That's why weighing yourself daily is as important during Metabolic Adjustment as it was during your weight loss. When you step on the scale every morning, you'll know exactly where you stand.

If, during Metabolic Adjustment, you find it difficult to stay within the 1½-pound guideline, you're probably either eating too much of your menu foods, eating food that's not included on this phase of the program, and/or not exercising enough to burn the number of calories you're consuming. Review your Daily Action Plan to make sure you're consuming enough protein and that you're effectively controlling the amount of fat and refined carbohydrates you're eating. And, as always, monitor your level of activity.

Your success will come faster and easier if you resist the urge to alter the program in any way. Tens of thousands of people have learned to become Lean for Life *by following the program through all three phases*. It works! Eat all three meals—including all of the food additions specified on your program—even if you're "not hungry." (If you don't eat them, you soon will be.)

You've already succeeded in losing weight during the first phase of your program. Once your metabolism is elevated, you'll be ready to

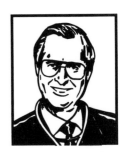

DR. STAMPER

"Remember to weigh yourself daily and correct for any 1½-pound gain. Do not move on to the next level of food additions until you have completed each level without a weight gain."

Your Turn

Staying motivated during the weight-loss phase of the program is easy because every day you see and feel the benefits. You "see the reward." *Staying motivated to maintain your weight, however, is more of a challenge.* You don't get to see or feel the progress.

That's why it's important for you to decide what your personal rewards for maintaining your weight loss "look like." In other words, what are the payoffs you are enjoying as a result of your maintaining your weight loss? By clearly identifying the specific benefits, you'll be more likely to sustain your motivation.

The following list includes a sampling of the benefits Lindora patients have described for maintaining their weight loss:

- ❑ "I can wear my favorite clothes without holding my stomach in."
- ❑ "I can run, bend, and jump without excess fat getting in the way."
- ❑ "For the first time in 10 years, both my blood pressure and cholesterol levels are normal."
- ❑ "I can tie my shoes without getting short of breath."
- ❑ "I no longer feel self-conscious about my body when I go to the beach."
- ❑ "My arthritis doesn't flare up as often because I'm not putting as much stress on my joints."
- ❑ "I recently had a physical and my doctor told me I'm in better shape now than I was four years ago."
- ❑ "I look and feel healthier than I did in college."

What "rewards" are you enjoying now that you've lost weight? Ask friends and family if they've noticed any other perks. You'll probably be surprised by what they say. List all the benefits and payoffs that come to mind:

_____

_____

_____

Update and review this list every day during Phase 2. Focusing on the benefits of maintaining your weight loss will motivate and remind you that *maintaining* is as important as losing.

either begin another weight-loss series or move into the final phase: Lifetime Maintenance.

SUCCESS STRATEGIES: 12 WAYS TO GUARANTEE RESULTS DURING METABOLIC ADJUSTMENT

During the Metabolic Adjustment phase of your program, it's important that you:

1. *Eat three meals a day.* We've already discussed why it's so vital to make all your Phase 2 food additions as outlined on your program. It's equally important that you eat three meals a day, every day. Because you've become used to eating less during your weight-loss phase, you may find yourself tempted to occasionally skip meals. Don't do it! You need to continue to reinforce the healthy patterns that you established during weight loss.

2. *Maintain your Daily Action Plan.* Your Daily Action Plan will help you stay aware of what, when, where, why, and how much you're eating. Be sure to keep a written record of your food during Phase 2. That way, if you experience any weight gain, you can review your record to determine what happened and know how to correct it.

3. *Weigh yourself each morning.* Continue this important habit.

4. *Listen to your tapes.* Every time you do, you'll discover new insights about the program—and yourself.

5. *Practice your affirmations.* The goal, of course, is to stay motivated and focused on reinforcing your healthy self-image.

6. *Exercise and monitor the number of steps you take.* There are countless physical and psychological payoffs to gentle exercise: It increases your mitochondria, elevates your mood, boosts your metabolism, burns calories, tones and firms your body, and helps you feel more relaxed and less hungry. Continue to use your "Warming Up" videotape, and walk or do some other form of gentle exercise at least five days a week.

7. *Take your vitamin and mineral supplements.* Since you'll be eating more food during this phase of your program, you only need to take one vitamin and mineral supplement with each meal.

8. *Do one Protein Day every week.* We recommend a weekly Protein Day during Phase 2 because it helps control your appetite and provides a structure of self-discipline that will benefit you as you move

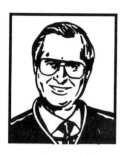

DR. STAMPER

"During Lifetime

Maintenance, it's

important to

continue doing

those things that

helped you *become*

Lean for Life."

toward Lifetime Maintenance. It's best to designate one day each week—preferably Monday—as your Protein Day. That way, you start your week off with a clear focus on your program and your progress.

9. *Drink at least 40 to 60 ounces of water or other calorie-free fluid every day.* Liquids—especially water—keep you hydrated, control appetite, and eliminate excess fluids. Although we encourage you to drink as much water as you can, you may reduce your liquid intake during "Phase 2: Metabolic Adjustment" to 40 to 60 ounces daily. You may continue to add lemon juice as desired.

10. *Avoid sugar, alcohol, hydrogenated fat, animal fats, and white flour.* Why? Here's a quick recap:

Sugar is not only loaded with empty calories, but it takes your system on a roller-coaster ride that ends with a dip in blood sugar and results in cravings.

When you eat sugar or high-carbohydrate foods, your body must produce insulin in the pancreas for you to utilize the concentrated carbohydrate calories. The insulin flows into your bloodstream to move the carbohydrates—which are now in the form of glucose—into the cells for use as energy. When this process occurs, your blood sugar drops. The result? You get hungry and crave carbohydrates. Protein, on the other hand, is metabolized more slowly, allowing your blood sugar to remain more stable and your appetite to remain in check. Your body doesn't need to produce insulin to utilize protein or fat. The bottom line: The less sugar you eat, the better off you'll be.

Alcohol not only contains empty calories, but it also inhibits self-control. If you choose to drink, stick with white wine or a wine spritzer. Caution: You may find that because you've avoided alcohol during the weight-loss phase of your program, you have a diminished tolerance and one drink now has the same effect as two or three. Be careful.

White flour and the baked goods that contain it are typically higher in carbohydrates and fat. Whole grains are healthier, and they taste better, too.

Hydrogenated fat and animal fats—butter, regular margarine, solid cooking fat, and coffee whiteners are artery cloggers loaded with unwanted calories. Choose unsaturated, nonhydrogenated fats, such as olive oil.

Having completed the weight-loss phase of your program, you've already reduced or eliminated these foods from your diet. You've taken some major steps forward. Why take even one step back?

11. *Use protein supplements, as needed, to control cravings.* Whenever you're overcome by a "snack attack," have a protein-enhanced snack and a large glass of water. Keep protein snacks handy—in your glove compartment, at work, in your purse, or pocket. That way, you always have a healthy choice available.

12. *Stay focused.* Phase 2 only takes two weeks. Stick with it—the results are worth it!

"MR. MITO" SAYS:

"The more you listen, the more you lose! Preliminary evidence from studies at the University of Wisconsin suggest that listening to motivational tapes can—and does—affect one's weight. In one study, participants raised their metabolic rates simply by listening to guided imagery tapes that helped them focus on revving up their metabolism."

ANY QUESTIONS?

Q: *Why should I care about Metabolic Adjustment? What's in it for me?*

A: No one ever goes on a weight-loss program believing "I'm going to lose 30 pounds and then gain it back!" They think "Once I lose the weight, I'll be fine—I'm never going to be fat again!"

But the truth is most people who diet—some experts suggest as many as 95%— regain all their weight within five years. That's why the focus of Lean for Life isn't simply on losing weight. It's maintaining your weight loss that ultimately makes the difference. *Metabolic Adjustment is a valuable and necessary phase in this process.*

Lean *for* Life®
DAILY ACTION PLAN

LEVEL I METABOLIC ADJUSTMENT

Week ___I___ Day ___I___ Date _____

Time	Meal Plans		Serving Size	Carbs (grams)
	Breakfast			
	Protein	2		
	Fruit or Grain	1 1/2		
	Beverage	1		
	Protein Snack			
	Lunch			
	Protein	1 1/2		
	Vegetable	1		
	Lettuce	Unl.		
	Fruit	1		
	Beverage	1		
	Miscellaneous	2		
	Protein Snack			
	Dinner			
	Protein	1 1/2		
	Vegetable	1		
	Lettuce	Unl.		
	Fruit	1		
	Beverage	1		
	Miscellaneous	2		
	Protein Snack			
			TOTAL	

Weight _____

Vitamins   AM   Noon   PM

Water _____

Activities _____
_____
_____
_____

\# Pedometer Steps _____

WEEKLY BODY MEASUREMENTS

Chest _____   Hips _____
Waist _____   Thighs _____
Abdomen _____

SUCCESS LEARNING TOOLS

Read pages # _____
Audio Tape _____
Video _____
CD-ROM _____
Bio-Card ™ _____
Affirmation _____

Other _____
Plan to Overcome Today's Obstacles:
_____
_____
_____
_____

Notes:
_____
_____
_____
_____
_____

CHOOSE ONE DAY EACH WEEK DURING METABOLIC ADJUSTMENT
AS YOUR "PROTEIN DAY." DO YOUR "PROTEIN DAY" EXACTLY
AS YOU DID DURING WEIGHT LOSS.

Lean *for* Life®
DAILY ACTION PLAN

LEVEL I METABOLIC ADJUSTMENT

Week ___I___   Day ___2___   Date _____

Time	Meal Plans	Serving Size	Carbs (grams)
	Breakfast		
	Protein	2	
	Fruit or Grain	1 1/2	
	Beverage	1	
	Protein Snack		
	Lunch		
	Protein	1 1/2	
	Vegetable	1	
	Lettuce	Unl.	
	Fruit	1	
	Beverage	1	
	Miscellaneous	2	
	Protein Snack		
	Dinner		
	Protein	1 1/2	
	Vegetable	1	
	Lettuce	Unl.	
	Fruit	1	
	Beverage	1	
	Miscellaneous	2	
	Protein Snack		
		TOTAL	

Weight _____

Vitamins ____ AM ____ Noon ____ PM ____

Water _____

Activities _____
_____
_____

\# Pedometer Steps _____

WEEKLY BODY MEASUREMENTS

Chest _____ Hips _____
Waist _____ Thighs _____
Abdomen _____

SUCCESS LEARNING TOOLS

Read pages # _____
Audio Tape _____
Video _____
CD-ROM _____
Bio-Card ™ _____
Affirmation _____
_____

Other _____
Plan to Overcome Today's Obstacles:
_____
_____
_____
_____
_____

Notes: _____
_____
_____
_____

CHOOSE ONE DAY EACH WEEK DURING METABOLIC ADJUSTMENT AS YOUR "PROTEIN DAY." DO YOUR "PROTEIN DAY" EXACTLY AS YOU DID DURING WEIGHT LOSS.

Lean *for* Life®
DAILY ACTION PLAN

LEVEL I METABOLIC ADJUSTMENT

Week ___I___ Day ___3___ Date _____

Time	Meal Plans		Serving Size	Carbs (grams)
	Breakfast			
	Protein	2		
	Fruit or Grain	1 1/2		
	Beverage	1		
	Protein Snack			
	Lunch			
	Protein	1 1/2		
	Vegetable	1		
	Lettuce	Unl.		
	Fruit	1		
	Beverage	1		
	Miscellaneous	2		
	Protein Snack			
	Dinner			
	Protein	1 1/2		
	Vegetable	1		
	Lettuce	Unl.		
	Fruit	1		
	Beverage	1		
	Miscellaneous	2		
	Protein Snack			
			TOTAL	

Weight

Vitamins	AM	Noon	PM

Water

Activities _____
_____
_____

Pedometer Steps

WEEKLY BODY MEASUREMENTS

Chest		Hips	
Waist		Thighs	
Abdomen			

SUCCESS LEARNING TOOLS

Read pages # _____
Audio Tape _____
Video _____
CD-ROM _____
Bio-Card ™ _____
Affirmation _____

Other _____
Plan to Overcome Today's Obstacles: _____
_____
_____
_____
_____

Notes: _____
_____
_____
_____

CHOOSE ONE DAY EACH WEEK DURING METABOLIC ADJUSTMENT AS YOUR "PROTEIN DAY." DO YOUR "PROTEIN DAY" EXACTLY AS YOU DID DURING WEIGHT LOSS.

Lean for Life®
DAILY ACTION PLAN

LEVEL 2 METABOLIC ADJUSTMENT

Week ___I___ Day ___4___ Date _____

Time	Meal Plans	Serving Size	Carbs (grams)
	Breakfast		
	Protein	2	
	Fruit or Grain	I 1/2	
	Beverage	I	
	Protein Snack		
	Lunch		
	Protein	2	
	Vegetable	I	
	Lettuce	Unl.	
	Fruit	I	
	Beverage	I	
	Miscellaneous	2	
	Protein Snack		
	Dinner		
	Protein	2	
	Vegetable	I	
	Lettuce	Unl.	
	Fruit	I	
	Beverage	I	
	Miscellaneous	2	
	Protein Snack		
		TOTAL	

Weight _____
Vitamins   AM   Noon   PM
Water _____

Activities _____

Pedometer Steps _____

WEEKLY BODY MEASUREMENTS

Chest _____   Hips _____
Waist _____   Thighs _____
Abdomen _____

SUCCESS LEARNING TOOLS

Read pages # _____
Audio Tape _____
Video _____
CD-ROM _____
Bio-Card ™ _____
Affirmation _____

Other _____
Plan to Overcome Today's Obstacles: _____

Notes: _____

CHOOSE ONE DAY EACH WEEK DURING METABOLIC ADJUSTMENT AS YOUR "PROTEIN DAY." DO YOUR "PROTEIN DAY" EXACTLY AS YOU DID DURING WEIGHT LOSS.

Lean *for* Life®
DAILY ACTION PLAN

LEVEL 2 METABOLIC ADJUSTMENT

Week ___I___ Day ___5___ Date _____

Time	Meal Plans	Serving Size	Carbs (grams)
	Breakfast		
	Protein	2	
	Fruit or Grain	1 1/2	
	Beverage	1	
	Protein Snack		
	Lunch		
	Protein	2	
	Vegetable	1	
	Lettuce	Unl.	
	Fruit	1	
	Beverage	1	
	Miscellaneous	2	
	Protein Snack		
	Dinner		
	Protein	2	
	Vegetable	1	
	Lettuce	Unl.	
	Fruit	1	
	Beverage	1	
	Miscellaneous	2	
	Protein Snack		
		TOTAL	

Weight
Vitamins   AM   Noon   PM
Water

Activities

Pedometer Steps

WEEKLY BODY MEASUREMENTS
Chest   Hips
Waist   Thighs
Abdomen

SUCCESS LEARNING TOOLS
Read pages #
Audio Tape
Video
CD-ROM
Bio-Card™
Affirmation

Other
Plan to Overcome Today's Obstacles:

Notes:

CHOOSE ONE DAY EACH WEEK DURING METABOLIC ADJUSTMENT AS YOUR "PROTEIN DAY." DO YOUR "PROTEIN DAY" EXACTLY AS YOU DID DURING WEIGHT LOSS.

Lean *for* Life®
DAILY ACTION PLAN

LEVEL 2 METABOLIC ADJUSTMENT

Week ___I___ Day ___6___ Date _____

Time	Meal Plans	Serving Size	Carbs (grams)
	Breakfast		
	Protein	2	
	Fruit or Grain	I 1/2	
	Beverage	I	
	Protein Snack		
	Lunch		
	Protein	2	
	Vegetable	I	
	Lettuce	Unl.	
	Fruit	I	
	Beverage	I	
	Miscellaneous	2	
	Protein Snack		
	Dinner		
	Protein	2	
	Vegetable	I	
	Lettuce	Unl.	
	Fruit	I	
	Beverage	I	
	Miscellaneous	2	
	Protein Snack		
		TOTAL	

Weight _____

Vitamins	AM	Noon	PM

Water _____

Activities _____

Pedometer Steps _____

WEEKLY BODY MEASUREMENTS

Chest _____ Hips _____
Waist _____ Thighs _____
Abdomen _____

SUCCESS LEARNING TOOLS

Read pages # _____
Audio Tape _____
Video _____
CD-ROM _____
Bio-Card ™ _____
Affirmation _____

Other _____
Plan to Overcome Today's Obstacles: _____

Notes: _____

CHOOSE ONE DAY EACH WEEK DURING METABOLIC ADJUSTMENT
AS YOUR "PROTEIN DAY." DO YOUR "PROTEIN DAY" EXACTLY
AS YOU DID DURING WEIGHT LOSS.

Lean *for* Life®
DAILY ACTION PLAN

LEVEL 2 METABOLIC ADJUSTMENT

Week ___1___ Day ___7___ Date _____

Time	Meal Plans		Serving Size	Carbs (grams)
	Breakfast			
	Protein	2		
	Fruit or Grain	1 1/2		
	Beverage	1		
	Protein Snack			
	Lunch			
	Protein	2		
	Vegetable	1		
	Lettuce	Unl.		
	Fruit	1		
	Beverage	1		
	Miscellaneous	2		
	Protein Snack			
	Dinner			
	Protein	2		
	Vegetable	1		
	Lettuce	Unl.		
	Fruit	1		
	Beverage	1		
	Miscellaneous	2		
	Protein Snack			
			TOTAL	

Weight _____

Vitamins	AM	Noon	PM

Water _____

Activities _____

Pedometer Steps _____

WEEKLY BODY MEASUREMENTS

Chest _____ Hips _____
Waist _____ Thighs _____
Abdomen _____

SUCCESS LEARNING TOOLS

Read pages # _____
Audio Tape _____
Video _____
CD-ROM _____
Bio-Card™ _____
Affirmation _____

Other _____
Plan to Overcome Today's Obstacles: _____

Notes: _____

CHOOSE ONE DAY EACH WEEK DURING METABOLIC ADJUSTMENT
AS YOUR "PROTEIN DAY." DO YOUR "PROTEIN DAY" EXACTLY
AS YOU DID DURING WEIGHT LOSS.

Lean for Life®
DAILY ACTION PLAN

LEVEL 3 METABOLIC ADJUSTMENT

Week __2__ Day __8__ Date _____

Time	Meal Plans	Serving Size	Carbs (grams)
____	**Breakfast**		
	Protein	2	
	Fruit or Grain	1 1/2	
	Beverage	1	
____	**Protein Snack**		
____	**Lunch**		
	Protein	2	
	Vegetable	1	
	Lettuce	Unl.	
	Fruit	1	
	Grain	1	
	Beverage	1	
	Miscellaneous	2	
____	**Protein Snack**		
____	**Dinner**		
	Protein	2	
	Vegetable	1	
	Lettuce	Unl.	
	Fruit	1	
	Grain	1	
	Beverage	1	
	Miscellaneous	2	
____	**Protein Snack**		
		TOTAL	

Weight _____

Vitamins   AM   Noon   PM _____

Water _____

Activities _____

\# Pedometer Steps _____

WEEKLY BODY MEASUREMENTS

Chest _____	Hips _____
Waist _____	Thighs _____
Abdomen _____	

SUCCESS LEARNING TOOLS

Read pages # _____

Audio Tape _____

Video _____

CD-ROM _____

Bio-Card ™ _____

Affirmation _____

Other _____

Plan to Overcome Today's Obstacles:

_____

_____

_____

Notes:

_____

_____

CHOOSE ONE DAY EACH WEEK DURING METABOLIC ADJUSTMENT AS YOUR "PROTEIN DAY." DO YOUR "PROTEIN DAY" EXACTLY AS YOU DID DURING WEIGHT LOSS.

Lean *for* Life®
DAILY ACTION PLAN

LEVEL 3 METABOLIC ADJUSTMENT

Week __2__   Day __9__   Date _____

Time	Meal Plans	Serving Size	Carbs (grams)
	Breakfast		
	Protein	2	
	Fruit or Grain	1 1/2	
	Beverage	1	
	Protein Snack		
	Lunch		
	Protein	2	
	Vegetable	1	
	Lettuce	Unl.	
	Fruit	1	
	Grain	1	
	Beverage	1	
	Miscellaneous	2	
	Protein Snack		
	Dinner		
	Protein	2	
	Vegetable	1	
	Lettuce	Unl.	
	Fruit	1	
	Grain	1	
	Beverage	1	
	Miscellaneous	2	
	Protein Snack		
		TOTAL	

Weight _____

Vitamins   AM _____   Noon _____   PM _____

Water _____

Activities _____

Pedometer Steps _____

WEEKLY BODY MEASUREMENTS

Chest _____   Hips _____

Waist _____   Thighs _____

Abdomen _____

SUCCESS LEARNING TOOLS

Read pages # _____

Audio Tape _____

Video _____

CD-ROM _____

Bio-Card ™ _____

Affirmation _____

Other _____

Plan to Overcome Today's Obstacles:

_____

_____

_____

Notes:

_____

_____

_____

CHOOSE ONE DAY EACH WEEK DURING METABOLIC ADJUSTMENT AS YOUR "PROTEIN DAY." DO YOUR "PROTEIN DAY" EXACTLY AS YOU DID DURING WEIGHT LOSS.

Lean for Life®
DAILY ACTION PLAN

LEVEL 3 METABOLIC ADJUSTMENT

Week __2__ Day __10__ Date _____

Time	Meal Plans	Serving Size	Carbs (grams)
____	**Breakfast**		
	Protein	2	
	Fruit or Grain	1 1/2	
	Beverage	1	
____	**Protein Snack**		
____	**Lunch**		
	Protein	2	
	Vegetable	1	
	Lettuce	Unl.	
	Fruit	1	
	Grain	1	
	Beverage	1	
	Miscellaneous	2	
____	**Protein Snack**		
____	**Dinner**		
	Protein	2	
	Vegetable	1	
	Lettuce	Unl.	
	Fruit	1	
	Grain	1	
	Beverage	1	
	Miscellaneous	2	
____	**Protein Snack**		
		TOTAL	

Weight _____
Vitamins   AM _____   Noon _____   PM _____
Water _____

Activities _____
_____
_____
_____

Pedometer Steps _____

WEEKLY BODY MEASUREMENTS
Chest _____   Hips _____
Waist _____   Thighs _____
Abdomen _____

SUCCESS LEARNING TOOLS
Read pages # _____
Audio Tape _____
Video _____
CD-ROM _____
Bio-Card™ _____
Affirmation _____

Other _____
Plan to Overcome Today's Obstacles: _____
_____
_____
_____
_____

Notes: _____
_____
_____
_____

CHOOSE ONE DAY EACH WEEK DURING METABOLIC ADJUSTMENT
AS YOUR "PROTEIN DAY." DO YOUR "PROTEIN DAY" EXACTLY
AS YOU DID DURING WEIGHT LOSS.

Lean *for* Life®
DAILY ACTION PLAN

LEVEL 3 METABOLIC ADJUSTMENT

Week __2__   Day __II__   Date _____

Time	Meal Plans	Serving Size	Carbs (grams)
	Breakfast		
	Protein	2	
	Fruit or Grain	1 1/2	
	Beverage	1	
	Protein Snack		
	Lunch		
	Protein	2	
	Vegetable	1	
	Lettuce	Unl.	
	Fruit	1	
	Grain	1	
	Beverage	1	
	Miscellaneous	2	
	Protein Snack		
	Dinner		
	Protein	2	
	Vegetable	1	
	Lettuce	Unl.	
	Fruit	1	
	Grain	1	
	Beverage	1	
	Miscellaneous	2	
	Protein Snack		
		TOTAL	

Weight _____

Vitamins	AM	Noon	PM

Water _____

Activities _____

\# Pedometer Steps _____

WEEKLY BODY MEASUREMENTS

Chest	Hips
Waist	Thighs
Abdomen	

SUCCESS LEARNING TOOLS

Read pages # _____
Audio Tape _____
Video _____
CD-ROM _____
Bio-Card™ _____
Affirmation _____

Other _____
Plan to Overcome Today's Obstacles: _____

Notes: _____

CHOOSE ONE DAY EACH WEEK DURING METABOLIC ADJUSTMENT AS YOUR "PROTEIN DAY." DO YOUR "PROTEIN DAY" EXACTLY AS YOU DID DURING WEIGHT LOSS.

Lean *for* Life®
DAILY ACTION PLAN

LEVEL 3 METABOLIC ADJUSTMENT

Week __2__   Day __12__   Date _____

Time	Meal Plans	Serving Size	Carbs (grams)
	Breakfast		
	Protein	2	
	Fruit or Grain	1 1/2	
	Beverage	1	
	Protein Snack		
	Lunch		
	Protein	2	
	Vegetable	1	
	Lettuce	Unl.	
	Fruit	1	
	Grain	1	
	Beverage	1	
	Miscellaneous	2	
	Protein Snack		
	Dinner		
	Protein	2	
	Vegetable	1	
	Lettuce	Unl.	
	Fruit	1	
	Grain	1	
	Beverage	1	
	Miscellaneous	2	
	Protein Snack		
		TOTAL	

Weight _____
Vitamins   AM ____   Noon ____   PM ____
Water _____

Activities _____
_____
_____

Pedometer Steps _____

WEEKLY BODY MEASUREMENTS
Chest _____   Hips _____
Waist _____   Thighs _____
Abdomen _____

SUCCESS LEARNING TOOLS
Read pages # _____
Audio Tape _____
Video _____
CD-ROM _____
Bio-Card™ _____
Affirmation _____

Other _____
Plan to Overcome Today's Obstacles: _____
_____
_____
_____
_____

Notes: _____
_____
_____
_____

CHOOSE ONE DAY EACH WEEK DURING METABOLIC ADJUSTMENT AS YOUR "PROTEIN DAY." DO YOUR "PROTEIN DAY" EXACTLY AS YOU DID DURING WEIGHT LOSS.

Lean *for* Life®
DAILY ACTION PLAN

LEVEL 3 METABOLIC ADJUSTMENT

Week __2__ Day __13__ Date _____

Time	Meal Plans	Serving Size	Carbs (grams)
	Breakfast		
	Protein	2	
	Fruit or Grain	1 1/2	
	Beverage	1	
	Protein Snack		
	Lunch		
	Protein	2	
	Vegetable	1	
	Lettuce	Unl.	
	Fruit	1	
	Grain	1	
	Beverage	1	
	Miscellaneous	2	
	Protein Snack		
	Dinner		
	Protein	2	
	Vegetable	1	
	Lettuce	Unl.	
	Fruit	1	
	Grain	1	
	Beverage	1	
	Miscellaneous	2	
	Protein Snack		
		TOTAL	

Weight _____

Vitamins   AM _____   Noon _____   PM _____

Water _____

Activities _____
_____
_____
_____

Pedometer Steps _____

WEEKLY BODY MEASUREMENTS

Chest _____   Hips _____
Waist _____   Thighs _____
Abdomen _____

SUCCESS LEARNING TOOLS

Read pages # _____
Audio Tape _____
Video _____
CD-ROM _____
Bio-Card™ _____
Affirmation _____

Other _____
Plan to Overcome Today's Obstacles: _____
_____
_____
_____
_____
_____

Notes: _____
_____
_____
_____
_____

CHOOSE ONE DAY EACH WEEK DURING METABOLIC ADJUSTMEN'
AS YOUR "PROTEIN DAY." DO YOUR "PROTEIN DAY" EXACTLY
AS YOU DID DURING WEIGHT LOSS.

Lean for Life®
DAILY ACTION PLAN

LEVEL 3 METABOLIC ADJUSTMENT

Week __2__   Day __14__   Date _____

Time	Meal Plans	Serving Size	Carbs (grams)	
	Breakfast			
	Protein	2		
	Fruit or Grain	1 1/2		
	Beverage	1		
	Protein Snack			
	Lunch			
	Protein	2		
	Vegetable	1		
	Lettuce	Unl.		
	Fruit	1		
	Grain	1		
	Beverage	1		
	Miscellaneous	2		
	Protein Snack			
	Dinner			
	Protein	2		
	Vegetable	1		
	Lettuce	Unl.		
	Fruit	1		
	Grain	1		
	Beverage	1		
	Miscellaneous	2		
	Protein Snack			
		TOTAL		

Weight _____
Vitamins   AM _____   Noon _____   PM _____
Water _____

Activities _____
_____
_____

Pedometer Steps _____

WEEKLY BODY MEASUREMENTS
Chest _____   Hips _____
Waist _____   Thighs _____
Abdomen _____

SUCCESS LEARNING TOOLS
Read pages # _____
Audio Tape _____
Video _____
CD-ROM _____
Bio-Card™ _____
Affirmation _____

Other _____
Plan to Overcome Today's Obstacles:
_____
_____
_____
_____
_____

Notes:
_____
_____
_____
_____

CHOOSE ONE DAY EACH WEEK DURING METABOLIC ADJUSTMENT
AS YOUR "PROTEIN DAY." DO YOUR "PROTEIN DAY" EXACTLY
AS YOU DID DURING WEIGHT LOSS.

8

"PHASE 3: LIFETIME MAINTENANCE"

You'll discover how to stabilize at your new lean weight so you can eat normally without regaining weight

Imagine, if you will, a weight-loss program called "The Amazing Yo-Yo Diet." On it, you would lose all the weight you wanted. You would look terrific and feel fabulous. People would compliment you on your success.

Then, within days of achieving your goal, you would gradually begin regaining the weight—a pound here, a half-pound there. Over time, the sense of pride and accomplishment you initially felt would be eclipsed by disappointment and disbelief as you realized you had gained back every single pound you'd lost.

Sounds more like an exercise in frustration and futility than an effective approach to weight loss, doesn't it? Yet that's exactly what millions of people do every year. Studies show that more than 95% of those who complete weight-loss programs regain their weight within five years. Why? Because instead of embracing their success by learning how to maintain their lean weight, they revert back to the habits that made them fat in the first place. By committing to *losing* weight but not to *keeping it off,* they win the battle but lose the war.

It doesn't have to be that way. This program is called Lean for Life for good reason. It not only helps you lose weight, it shows you how you can

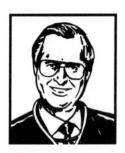

DR. STAMPER

"If you find yourself regaining weight, skip your evening meal and have only the protein portion. Take charge. Take control."

maintain your new lean weight for life! Follow the Lean for Life program through "Phase 3: Lifetime Maintenance" and you'll never need to diet again.

THE CHALLENGE

Lifetime maintenance is more than a phase of a weight-control program. It's a mindset and an attitude. It's about taking care of yourself and making healthy choices. It's an on-going, day-by-day process of recommitting yourself to the excellence you've achieved. During the first three to six months of "Phase 3: Lifetime Maintenance," you will gradually add a variety of foods to your diet to determine how much your body can tolerate without a weight gain, all while continuing to practice the success strategies you learned during the weight-loss phase of the program.

Many people find "Phase 3: Lifetime Maintenance" to be the most challenging part of the program. Some don't fully appreciate the value and benefits of this final phase. Their "urgency factor" is no longer quite so urgent. And since they're feeling healthier and more attractive, the need to do the work necessary to maintain often doesn't seem as pressing as their need to lose weight did just weeks earlier. On the heels of their recent success, it's easy to persuade themselves they've been "cured"—that they've "done it" and are finally "over the hump." Unfortunately, the value of—and the need for—"Phase 3: Lifetime Maintenance" often doesn't become apparent until it's too late.

If you want to maintain your weight loss, you must maintain the behavior change that made it happen. That's exactly what "Phase 3: Lifetime Maintenance" is designed to help you do. Like the earlier phases of the program, it has been revised, refined, and perfected over 25 years. It works! Thousands of Lindora patients who have lost weight on other programs, only to gain it all back, have successfully maintained their weight loss by practicing the basic principles of this third phase. You can, too.

STABILIZING AT YOUR NEW LEAN WEIGHT

During "Phase 3: Lifetime Maintenance," your goal is simple and specific—to stabilize at your new lean weight so that you will be able to eat normally without gaining weight. This is a crucial step because even after you've reached your lean weight, your body's setpoint remains elevated. If you begin eating the way you have in the past, you will very likely regain the weight just as rapidly as you lost it.

In order to stabilize your body at your new lean weight, it's critical that you maintain your weight within three pounds long enough to allow the weight-regulating center in your hypothalamus to accept your new weight as "normal" and to make adjustments in the metabolic feedback system we discussed back on Day 4. This, in turn, helps to reset your setpoint.

Remember when we likened the setpoint to a thermostat? When you're overweight, your setpoint adjusts upward to accommodate your body's increased caloric needs. When you lose weight, you need to adjust your setpoint downward so that it doesn't set off those annoying metabolic "alarm bells"—the ones that lead to cravings, urges to overeat, overeating, weight gain, and that maddening cycle known as "yo-yo dieting."

ACHIEVING EQUILIBRIUM

The process of resetting your setpoint and stabilizing your weight typically takes three to six months. After three months, you can determine whether you've stabilized at your new weight and reached equilibrium. Equilibrium is a state in which your weight has stabilized and your setpoint has readjusted, making it possible for you to eat more while still maintaining your lean weight.

How will you know whether you've achieved equilibrium? By eating a "test meal," a large evening meal of balanced food groups that is larger than you are accustomed to eating. How much larger depends on how much you're currently eating. A 200-pound man, for example, can eat—and therefore add—more food than a 100-pound woman. If your body has reached equilibrium at its new lean weight, your weight will stay approximately the same, even after your "test meal."

If you do gain, you'll know your body has not yet stabilized at its new weight. If this happens, you'll need to get back to your lean weight by having only protein for your evening meals until you lose the weight you've regained. Once you've done that, your goal then becomes to stay within three pounds of your lean weight for another three to four weeks. Then try again with another test meal until you can eat it without gaining weight.

Once your body has stabilized at its lean weight, you'll find you can eat more food—within reason—and not gain weight. But because your body may always be sensitive to large quantities of carbohydrates and fats, you may never be able to resume your old eating habits without a weight gain. You will, however, be able to eat generous amounts of healthy foods—and occasionally even splurge—and still stay Lean for Life.

LEAN FOODS VS. FAT FOODS

At Lindora, we encourage patients beginning "Phase 3: Lifetime Maintenance" to think of foods in two categories: Lean Foods and Fat Foods.

Lean foods contain less than 30% fat calories and are low or moderate in simple carbohydrates. These foods—especially those with

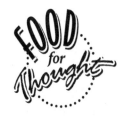

"There are plenty of alibis for failure. Success doesn't need them."

— Anonymous

WHAT STRESS CAN DO TO YOUR BODY AND YOUR BRAIN

It's no secret that stress takes its toll on the human body. It can cause a variety of health problems ranging from hives and headaches to severe muscle tension, stomach disorders, and even weight gain resulting from "stress eating."

Some experts are more convinced than ever that sustained stress can also wreak havoc on—and in—your brain, too. A study published in the August 1996 issue of *Science* reports that brain scans (MRI's) performed on people who have endured long-term stress during combat or childhood abuse show a significant decrease in the size of certain parts of their brains, providing compelling evidence of the connection between our minds and bodies.

So make a point to continue practicing your stress management skills. They'll not only ease the pressure and help you stay Lean for Life, but your brain will be healthier, too!

less than 15% fat calories—are the foundation for maintaining your new lean weight. Lean foods also include fruits, vegetables, and grains prepared with no (or very low) amounts of fat and sugar.

Foods with 20% to 30% fat calories are to be eaten as tolerated. This means that as you begin reintroducing these higher fat foods—and especially higher carbohydrate foods—into your daily diet, you'll need to pay close attention to how your body metabolizes them. If you find you're gradually gaining weight, you'll know that you're sensitive to these foods and must eat them less often.

Fat foods contain more than 30% fat calories. Foods that are high in calories from carbs or fat and low in nutritional value also fall into this category. Eat too much "fat food" such as candy, cookies, junk food, and fast food, and you will gain weight. If you're not careful, you can easily consume more calories in a single meal of fat foods than your body needs for an entire day. Review the section on how to read food labels on page 182.

If you do choose to eat fat foods, be aware of how much and how often you're eating them. Set limits. Remember that the fat you eat is the fat you wear. Eating well—and staying Lean for Life—is a choice you will need to make every day. Ultimately, how you eat, what you eat, and when you eat is up to you. The choice is always yours.

"SO WHAT DO I EAT?"

Over the next three to six months as you stabilize at your new lean weight, you'll be following the same basic food plan, but with one big difference—you'll be consuming more choices. In addition to the menu choices available during "Phase One: Weight Loss," you'll also be eating other healthy foods. Your daily menu consists of:

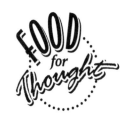

"The greatest freedom you have is the freedom to discipline yourself."

— Bernard Baruch

PROTEINS
3 daily servings (one per meal)

Your choice of one serving (average 100-200 calories each) at breakfast, lunch, and dinner. Be sure to weigh meat, seafood, and poultry after removing any skin, bone, and visible fat. Broil, boil, barbecue, microwave, roast, or "fry" using Pam spray or an equivalent. Your healthiest choice are high-protein foods that are lowest in fat and calories. Read labels on canned or packaged proteins carefully.

VEGETABLES
At least two daily servings

Choose at least two servings (average 40 calories each) a day, one each at lunch and dinner. Lettuce and other leafy greens? Have all you want. Measure vegetables raw, frozen (thawed), or water packed (drained). Read labels on packaged food for exact calories.

GRAINS
3 servings (men may tolerate more)

Choose three servings a day (average 100 calories each) of bread, rice, pasta, crackers, and cereals, as tolerated. This simply means that if you find yourself regaining weight, eliminate one grain serving. Remember that grains are high in carbohydrates, so choose accordingly. Limit dry cereals to one cup and cooked cereals to 3/4 cup per serving. Note that the percentage of fat in snack crackers varies between 30% to 50% or more. Choose low-fat or nonfat crackers that don't exceed 30% fat.

FRUITS
3 daily servings (one per meal)

Your choice of three servings (average 90 calories each), incuding at least one citrus fruit every day. Choose fresh, frozen (thawed), or water packed, with no sugar or juice added.

FAT
3 servings

Choose three servings a day (average 100 calories each). Remember that fat has nine calories per gram—more than double the number of calories per gram of carbohydrates or protein. Be sure to limit your fat calories to no more than 30%. Again, read labels carefully—while Fat Free Promise Ultra Light and Fleischmann's Non-Fat Margarine have just five calories per serving, most other "diet" and "light" margarines are 100% calories from fat. Since most foods contain some fat, you need to pay close attention to what you're eating to make sure that fat doesn't "sneak" into your diet and back on to your body. Before you eat it, ask yourself, "Is it worth it?"

SNACKS
3 protein choices per day

Continue the habit of mid-morning, mid-afternoon, and evening snacks—and continue to make them proteins!

MISCELLANEOUS
Unlimited

Be sure to count the calories of all miscellaneous foods. Miscellaneous foods include any items that are five calories per serving or less.

DESSERT
(Optional: One daily serving; counts as either a grain or fruit serving)

Dessert? In a "diet book"? That's right! Now that you've gotten down to your lean weight, you have choices that wouldn't have been productive during weight loss. One of them is the option of having a four-ounce serving of fat-free ice cream or frozen yogurt containing 90 calories or less as a substitution for one of your daily fruit or grain servings. You can also try low-fat ice cream, but steer clear of any that have more than 30% fat or more than 100 calories per four-ounce serving.

Notice that all your meals are based on protein, just as they were during the weight-loss phase of the program. Be sure to eat all your protein servings to avoid becoming hungry and to help control cravings. Now that you've achieved your lean weight, there's more flexibility in your plan as to what you eat and when you eat it. If, for example, you have two grain servings at lunch and none at dinner, it's not going to affect your weight. But if you start having two at lunch and one or two at dinner, you'll probably begin noticing a gradual weight increase. Watch out for this. Also be sure to start your day with a healthy breakfast. Breakfast-skippers invariably end up becoming night-time snackers.

It's a good idea to buy a food content book—they're available in paperback—that lists the calories, protein, carbohydrate, and fat content in thousands of foods. Remember that you'll no longer be

"HOW MUCH CAN I EAT?"

WOMEN

Active (6,000 steps or more per day on pedometer)
12-14 calories per pound of body weight

Weight	Calories per day	45% Carbohydrates 4 cal= 1 gram Calories (grams)	25% Protein 4 cal=1 gram Calories (grams)	30% Fat (or less) 9 cal=1 gram Calories (grams)
100 lb.	1,200-1,400	540-630 (135-158)	300-350 (75-88)	360-420 (40-47)
120 lb.	1,440-1,680	648-756 (162-189)	360-420 (90-105)	432-504 (48-56)
140 lb.	1,680-1,960	756-882 (189-221)	420-490 (105-123)	504-588 (56-65)
160 lb.	1,920-2,240	864-1,008 (216-252)	480-560 (120-140)	576-672 (64-75)

Inactive (5,000 steps or less per day on pedometer)
10-12 calories per pound of body weight

Weight	Calories per day	Calories (grams)	Calories (grams)	Calories (grams)
100 lb.	1,000-1,200	450-540 (113-135)	250-300 (63-75)	300-360 (33-40)
120 lb.	1,200-1,440	540-648 (135-162)	300-360 (75-90)	360-432 (40-48)
140 lb.	1,400-1,680	630-756 (158-189)	350-420 (88-105)	420-504 (47-56)
160 lb.	1,600-1,920	720-864 (180-216)	400-480 (100-120)	480-576 (53-64)

MEN

Active (6,000 steps or more per day on pedometer)
14-16 calories per pound of body weight

Weight	Calories per day	45% Carbohydrates 4 cal= 1 gram Calories (grams)	25% Protein 4 cal=1 gram Calories (grams)	30% Fat (or less) 9 cal=1 gram Calories (grams)
150 lb.	2,100-2,400	945-1,080 (236-270)	525-600 (131-150)	630-720 (70-80)
170 lb.	2,380-2,720	1,071-1,224(268-306)	595-680 (149-170)	714-816 (79-91)
190 lb.	2,660-3,040	1,197-1,368(299-342)	665-760 (166-190)	798-912 (89-101)
210 lb.	2,940-3,360	1,323-1,512(331-378)	735-840 (184-210)	882-1,008 (98-112)

Inactive (5,000 steps or less per day on pedometer)
12-14 calories per pound of body weight

Weight	Calories per day	Calories (grams)	Calories (grams)	Calories (grams)
150 lb.	1,800-2,100	810-945 (203-236)	450-525 (113-131)	540-630 (60-70)
170 lb.	2,040-2,380	918-1,071 (230-268)	510-595 (128-149)	612-714 (68-79)
190 lb.	2,280-2,660	1,026-1,197 (257-299)	570-665 (143-166)	684-798 (76-89)
210 lb.	2,520-2,940	1,134-1,323 (284-331)	630-735 (158-184)	756-882 (84-98)

FAT-BUSTERS: EASY WAYS TO REDUCE YOUR FAT INTAKE

❑ Bake, braise, broil, roast, barbecue, or microwave all meats, fish and poultry. No frying.
❑ Steam vegetables in a little water, then add herbs and lemon instead of butter.
❑ Choose nonfat margarines and spreads. There are a number of new ones on the market.
❑ Choose whole grain breads and pasta instead of those made with refined white flour.
❑ Limit your consumption of red meats. Choose turkey, chicken, and fish.
❑ Trim all visible fat and skin from meats and poultry.
❑ Make salad dressings from nonfat yogurt and nonfat mayonnaise. Try bottled nonfat, low-calorie dressings.
❑ Substitute nonfat or low-fat cheese for the high-fat, high-calorie variety.
❑ Stir-fry fresh vegetables in bouillon.
❑ Read labels carefully to determine how many of the calories are from fat. Choose accordingly.

counting carbohydrates since you won't be in ketosis. You will, however, want to keep close tabs on how much you're eating and the carbs, protein, and fat it contains.

"HOW MUCH DO I EAT?"

How much food you'll be able to eat without gaining weight depends on a number of factors, including your gender, current weight, and level of activity.

An inactive 140-pound woman, for example, typically needs only 10 to 12 calories per pound of body weight to maintain her weight—somewhere in the neighborhood of 1,400 to 1,680 calories. An active 190-pound man, on the other hand, may be able to consume 14 to 16 calories per pound of body weight—2,660 and 3,040 calories—without gaining weight.

The chart on page 235 will help you estimate how many calories your body needs to maintain your present weight. It will also help you plan meals to ensure that you achieve a healthy balance of 45% carbohydrates, 25% protein, and 30% or less in fat. What's more, it helps you easily estimate how many grams of protein, carbohydrates, and fat you need.

To maximize your results, restrict your fat grams even more—35 to 45 grams for women, and 45 to 60 grams for men. The calories you "save" can then be used for either more protein or more healthy complex carbohydrates. Over time, you'll learn what works best for you. If you find yourself feeling hungry and rummaging through the cupboards for food when you know you've eaten enough, take a good look at what you've eaten during the day. You'll probably discover that you've eaten too many carbohydrates and not enough protein. As you know, eating protein will fill you up and satisfy your hunger, while eating carbohydrates will usually stimulate cravings and cause you to feel hungry. Each person is unique. Learn how your body reacts—and plan your food choices accordingly.

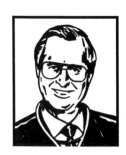

DR. STAMPER

"The strategies
that helped you
succeed in losing
weight will also
help you maintain
your weight."

SUCCESS STRATEGIES: 10 WAYS TO GUARANTEE RESULTS DURING "PHASE 3: LIFETIME MAINTENANCE"

Want to continue enjoying the benefits of being Lean for Life? Keep doing those things that helped you accomplish your weight-loss goal and you will!

1. *Maintain a support system*. This is especially important during the first three months of "Phase 3: Lifetime Maintenance." Whether you get support from friends, family members, at one of our clinics, or through the Lean for Life site on the World Wide Web, make a point to stay connected with people who appreciate what you've accomplished.

2. *Continue your gentle exercise*. This, too, must become a lifetime habit. Not only will exercise help you maintain your lean weight, but it also helps you control your appetite.

3. *Continue maintaining your Daily Action Plan until your weight has stabilized*. Behavior researchers report that people who are most successful at keeping their weight off are those who maintain a written record of their food and exercise. Whenever you find yourself regaining weight, keep a Daily Action Plan. It will help you regain awareness and regain control.

4. *Continue to weigh yourself every morning.* Make morning weigh-ins a lifetime habit. Addressing a minor weight gain today is much easier than being "surprised" by a 20-pound increase six months from now. Many successful maintainers tape their lean weight to their scale as a reminder. If you gain more than three pounds from your lean weight at any time during the first three months of "Phase 3: Lifetime Maintenance," have only protein for dinner until you've returned to your lean weight. Once you've stabilized your weight, do a Protein Day any time you gain more than three pounds. Take charge of the situation.

5. *Continue eating three meals a day.* This important pattern helps to program your mind and body when to eat. If you start eating whenever you decide you're "hungry" or whenever you "have time," odds are you'll end up snacking on whatever is handy rather than planning a healthy meal. When you do snack, think protein, fruits, and vegetables. Steer clear of high-carbohydrate snacks. Carbs can make you hungry if your body has difficulty metabolizing them.

6. *Continue doing one "Protein Day" every week.* This will help you maintain a sense of awareness and control over your eating, and will also help curb your appetite. Many successful maintainers choose Monday as their "Protein Day." This keeps them focused and in control as they begin each week. Some Lindora patients who have maintained their lean weight for more than 10 years find that when they begin each week with a protein breakfast and lunch—and then have a sensible dinner that evening—they can more easily control their appetite throughout the rest of the week.

7. *Continue drinking 40 to 60 ounces of calorie-free liquid every day.* This cleanses your system, helps curb appetite, and reduces fluid retention.

8. *Continue taking vitamins.* While you're probably eating healthier now than you ever have, one vitamin and mineral supplement with each meal helps insure that your body gets everything it needs to operate at peak efficiency.

9. *Continue to watch your caffeine and alcohol consumption.* Both can stimulate appetite—and alcohol contains empty calories. One shot of hard liquor totals around 100 calories.

10. *Continue doing your mental training exercises*. Mental training techniques such as affirmations, brief visualizations, and MENTORS Daily Mental Training sessions help focus your attention, adjust your energy level, and increase your confidence. These important tools helped get you where you are. They can also help you maintain your success.

THE 4 HABITS OF HIGHLY SUCCESSFUL MAINTAINERS

Why do some people succeed while others stumble? Over the years, the medical staff at Lindora has observed that virtually all successful maintainers exhibit four "habits" that clearly contribute to their success:

1. *Successful maintainers continue to practice the basics of the program*. You've just spent the past six weeks or more learning the basics and learning how to make them work for you. They helped get you this far—why would you abandon them now? On page 236, you'll find a list of 10 success strategies. Put them into action and you'll continue to be successful, too.

2. *Successful maintainers intentionally develop and maintain their self-image as a lean person*. How can you do the same? By making positive affirmations a part of your everyday life. By visualizing yourself as a thin person. By practicing an "achievement attitude" of optimism and positive problem-solving. You can use mental training techniques to experience yourself in particular situations, looking and feeling successful at your lean weight. You can avoid old patterns of overeating and inactivity.

3. *Successful maintainers are physically active*. How active do you need to be? Some people can maintain their weight by walking 30 minutes a day, while others need to walk more. The only way to determine how much activity is enough is to keep track of your exercise and see how it affects your weight. If you find that you're gaining weight even when you average 30 minutes of gentle exercise a day, see what happens if you increase it to 45 minutes. If your weight creeps up when you average 10,000 steps a day on your step counter, see what happens if you average 12,000 steps a day.

   Resolve to do whatever it takes. And remember, walking isn't your only option. As long as it's gentle, you can ride a bike, dance, swim, do water aerobics, in-line skate, ski, or use a variety of exercise machines at your local gym. One of the great benefits of becoming Lean for Life is that you've transformed yourself into an active person. Except for quitting smoking, this is the single most positive step a person can take to ensure lifetime good health.

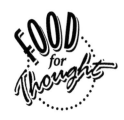

"Life is a mirror and will reflect back to the thinker what he thinks into it."

— Ernest Holmes

Your Turn

Take time to revisit the MENTORS Daily Mental Training exercise from Day 16 (page 143). It can help you focus on:

❑ resetting your setpoint to your new, leaner weight

❑ seeing yourself making healthy, appropriate food choices

❑ enjoying feeling enthused and energized while exercising

❑ increasing the strength and flexibility of your muscles

These tapes can be even more beneficial during Lifetime Maintenance. This type of mental training has been proven to be extremely effective. Did you know that nearly 100% of the athletes competing in the 1996 Summer Olympics engaged in some form of mental training? Let these proven techniques help you achieve your own "gold medal" in your quest to become—and stay—Lean for Life!

4. *Successful maintainers plan ahead for high-risk situations.* You and you alone are responsible for the choices you make. You can support yourself by anticipating challenges and developing a plan of action for managing potentially difficult situations. What will you do when a co-worker shows up with a platter of homemade brownies? When a snowstorm keeps you from walking outdoors? When you think ahead, you think more clearly—and react more effectively.

YOUR FUTURE—AND WELCOME TO IT!

Lifetime maintenance is clearly a journey rather than a destination. To paraphrase Anne Kaiser Stearns, whose wise words appear on one of the opening pages of this book, "If you keep doing what you've been doing, you'll keep getting the results you've gotten."

And if you don't, you won't. Any successful long-term maintainer will tell you that maintaining his or her lean weight requires determination, dedication, and discipline.

Remember Diana Rosenfeld, the Lean for Life ambassador whose inspiring story opened the first chapter of this book? Her numerous appearances on The Maury Povich Show and other television programs motivated people across the country to begin taking better care of themselves. Yet after losing 440 pounds in fewer than three years by applying the principles of the Lean for Life program, she began gradually reverting to habits that led to her weighing 640 pounds in the first place. The result? In 18 months, Diana regained nearly 25% of the weight she lost on the program.

Some might consider this a major setback or even a sign of failure. It's not necessarily either. It does, however, underscore the fact that obesity is a chronic condition. There is no such thing as a total cure. In order for Diana, you, or anyone else to lose weight and keep it off, it requires an investment in yourself. It takes focus, motivation, and an ongoing commitment to continue making appropriate, healthy choices.

The remarkable reality is that Diane has maintained a weight loss of more than 300 pounds for three years. Even more important, she possesses the knowledge, tools, and resources to reclaim her power, refocus her energy, and get back on track whenever she chooses.

And that, Diana says, is exactly what she's determined to do.

"I refuse to be a failure," she insists. "I'm too stubborn for that. This is not the end of the story. The story of Diana Rosenfeld is not over yet."

Your story isn't over, either. If you've just completed "Phase 2: Metabolic Adjustment" and are moving on to "Phase 3: Lifetime Maintenance," you've certainly ended a very positive chapter. Yet no matter how successful you've been in achieving your Lean for Life goal, remember that maintaining those results is ultimately what matters.

A year from now, how will your story read? Will you be a Lean for Life success story?

The choice, as always, is yours.

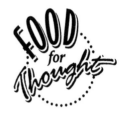

"Go confidently in the direction of your dreams. Live the life you have imagined."

— Henry David Thoreau

GLOSSARY

GLOSSARY

Affirmations

Positive statements that help establish patterns of desired actions and feelings.

Appetite

The desire to eat.

BioModification™

The act of intentionally changing your mental state in order to accomplish a specific purpose; also known as BioMod™

Body Composition Analysis

A procedure that measures the amount of fat, lean tissue, and water in the body.

Body Mass Index

A formula, based on height and weight, used to determine health risk factors and whether your weight is within a healthy or unhealthy range.

Chelation

A process that makes vitamins and minerals more absorbable by the body.

Cholesterol

A fatty substance produced in the liver and found in some foods.

Craving

A strong, nagging temptation for a particular food.

Daily Action Plan

A written record of food and activities designed to help you succeed on your weight-control program.

Defensive Barriers

The psychological defense mechanisms of denial and rationalization. Also known as internal barriers.

Denial

An unwillingness or refusal to admit or accept a reality.

Endorphins

Natural "feel good" hormones released in the body.

Food Withdrawal Symptoms

Temporary common physical symptoms, sometimes psychologically induced, that can occur when starting a weight-loss program.

Gallbladder Disease

Disease of the gallbladder that causes attacks of sharp pain in the upper right abdomen. Additional symptoms include nausea, gas, and bloating after eating. Common in people who are overweight.

Gentle Exercise

Exercise, such as walking, that doesn't cause breathlessness.

Inner Committee

Different aspects of your personality and temperament that sometimes cooperate and sometimes conflict.

Inner Dialogue

The ongoing discussion inside your mind.

Inner Mental Room

The place you create in your mind where you feel safe and can perform your mental training.

Insulin Receptors

Receptors on the surface of muscle cells that help move sugar into your muscles for active use instead of stored as fat.

Intentional Mental Activity

Techniques you do mentally to elicit an expected outcome.

Ketone Measuring Sticks or "Ketosticks"

Small plastic or paper strips used to measure the ketones excreted in your urine while on the weight-loss phase of the program. Also referred to as fat-burning indicators ("FBI").

Ketosis

The body's chemical state when body fat is being burned and used for energy; occurs during the first phase of the program.

"Lindorphins"

Lindora's name for endorphins, the "feel good" hormones released when you follow your weight-loss program and exercise.

Medical Grade Protein

High-grade, high-bioavailable protein.

Mental Blueprint

An intentional picture in your mind of yourself being the way you want to be and doing things in the way you want to do them.

Mental Training

A range of mental activities you can use to intentionally focus your attention, adjust your energy level, increase your confidence, or mentally practice specific actions.

MENTORS™ Daily Mental Training

A comprehensive program of audiocassette tapes and print materials created to guide you through daily sessions of calmness, focus, and mental rehearsal for the purpose of helping you reach and maintain your goals.

Metabolic Adjustment

The second phase of the Lean for Life program; a process of gradually increasing food intake while stabilizing body weight.

Metabolic Rate

The rate at which your body burns calories for energy.

Mind-Body Connection

A way of understanding the human organism that sees all aspects as united; when your thoughts affect your actions and your actions affect your thoughts.

Mitochondria

Tiny, egg-shaped structures in your cells that serve as fat-burning furnaces.

Motivator Cards

Written reminders of the benefits you'll enjoy when you've achieved your goal weight.

Mouth Hunger

The desire to eat and chew, even when you're not hungry.

Negative Self-Talk

A way of talking to yourself in disapproving, self-destructive language.

Orthostatic Hypotension

Low blood pressure resulting from a change in position.

Pavlovian Conditioning

The process of developing a particular response to a specific stimulus as a result of repeated reward.

Pedometer

A small measuring device that attaches to your belt or shoe and measures the number of steps taken; also known as a step counter.

Personal Satisfaction Quotient

A simple test to determine how you feel about your life at any given moment.

Pinch Test

An easy way to determine whether you have excess body fat.

Plateau

When you temporarily don't lose weight even though you're adhering to the program.

Prep Diet

A menu of foods eaten for one to three days before starting the program to insure healthy reserves of amino and fatty acids.

Protein Day

Days in which you eat protein-based foods; allows your body to achieve a state of ketosis more rapidly and is effective in controlling behavior and/or hunger.

Rationalizations

Excuses you make for your behavior.

Self-Awareness

Being conscious of your behavior and attitudes.

Self-Defeating Thoughts

Negative thinking that results in defeat.

Self-Esteem

A belief in your worth and value.

Self-Image

Your perception of yourself.

Setpoint or Settling Point

The weight at which your body's metabolic system seems to stabilize.

Skinny Mirror

A specially designed mirror in which your image appears thinner; a valuable tool in helping reinforce a thin mental image.

Synchronicity

Mind and body functioning in harmony.

Thought Control

Reframing your thoughts so they are helpful to you.

Urgency Factor

An incident, revelation, or "final straw" that motivates you to lose weight.

Vision Statement

A positive, short statement written in the present tense that describes how you see yourself looking, feeling, and acting in the future.

Visualization

The act of mentally experiencing yourself functioning better and being the way you desire, such as looking thinner, feeling healthier, eating less, and exercising more.

Willpower

The ability to resist temptation.

ABOUT THE AUTHORS

Cynthia Stamper Graff is president and chief executive officer of Lindora, Inc. She is also founder of the Lean for Life Foundation, a nonprofit organization that promotes obesity research and educational programs, and funds weight control services to selected low-income, morbidly obese men, women, and teenagers who meet the Foundation's financial criteria. An active participant in the growth and development of Lindora since 1972, she is nationally recognized as a leader in integrating technology into the treatment of obesity. She holds a law degree from York University in Toronto and lives in Newport Beach, California.

Jerry Holderman is an award-winning writer whose work has been featured in national magazines and syndicated in more than 60 North American newspapers, including the *Los Angeles Times, Washington Post, New York Post, Detroit News, Miami Herald, Chicago Sun-Times, Toronto Globe and Mail, Philadelphia Inquirer,* and *San Francisco Chronicle.* An honors graduate of the Oakland University School of Journalism, Rochester, Michigan, Holderman has collaborated on two other books and has worked as a video producer, entertainment publicist, radio feature reporter, speechwriter, and media consultant. Having lost 35 pounds on the program, he is a Lean for Life "success story." He lives in Los Angeles.

Lean for Life

for

Life

RESOURCES

A Message to Your Doctor

Your personal physician can be a valuable resource as you

do the Lean for Life program. We encourage you to

photocopy the following page from the book and give it

to your doctor so that he or she can easily contact Lindora's

executive medical director for additional information.

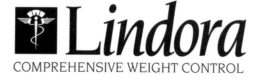

Dear Doctor:

As a physician who has dedicated his career to the treatment of obesity and its co-morbid medical conditions for more than twenty years, I understand how challenging the treatment of obesity can be.

I believe the scientifically sound, common sense approach of the Lean for Life program offers new hope and a strong, supportive structure to those people who desperately want—and need—to lose weight. This book is intended to be a therapeutic tool and treatment adjunct, to be used with your guidance to help your patient safely lose excess weight—and keep it off for life.

While *Lean for Life* provides your patient with a solid working knowledge of the science of fat loss, we at Lindora know that you—the physician who best knows the patient—are in a position to be his or her most valuable resource. There are a number of medications and medication combinations, for example, that may be appropriate adjunctive treatment for some patients, yet only after a professional assessment can such decisions be made. We have extensive experience with the use of medications and different prescription protocols that have proven to be effective.

I welcome the opportunity to be of service to you and your patients. If you would like to consult with me or receive more information on a medically supervised version of the Lean for Life program, please call or write to me at:

Lindora, Inc.
3505 Cadillac Avenue, Suite N-2
Costa Mesa, CA 92626
714/755-1157 x555

Sincerely,

Peter D. Vash, M.D., M.P.H.
Executive Medical Director, Lindora, Inc.
Assistant Clinical Professor, UCLA School of Medicine
Past President, American Society of Bariatric Physicians

"At Home, But Not Alone™"

To help you achieve the results you want,
we offer a number of support options:

A 24-hour **Telesupport System** is available to answer frequently asked questions (For example: What is ketosis? How fast will I lose weight? How do I get off this plateau? And more.)

1-900-225-LEAN

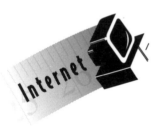

Visit our site on the **World Wide Web** and see "Breaking News" for the latest information in the weight loss field. Also try the "Ask The Expert" option where you can E-mail your questions to a physician trained in Bariatric Medicine.

www.leanforlife.com

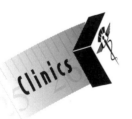

For a complete medically supervised program, visit any of the **Lindora Medical Clinics** located throughout Southern California.

1-800-LINDORA

Lindora Corporate Headquarters
3505 Cadillac Avenue, Suite N-2
Costa Mesa, CA 92626

From Friends of Lean for Life...

Following are special

products that the

Lindora medical staff

and members find

very beneficial

to their program

and their lives.

Lean for Life

PRODUCTS

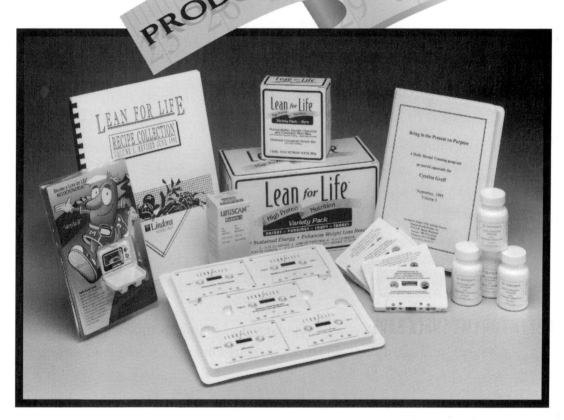

An assortment of products designed to enhance weight loss and weight maintenance results.

■ **STEP COUNTER:** Light, attractive, and fun to wear. Lindora patients rave about it and buy them for all their family members! A great way to be sure you're getting the exercise you need for the results you want!

■ **DR. STAMPER'S VITAMINS:** A formula developed specifically for the Lindora program.

■ **KETONE STRIPS:** Fat Burning Indicators (FBI!)

■ **AUDIO TAPES:** Developed to support the Lean for Life program.

■ **RECIPE BOOK:** Filled with simple, delicious recipes utilizing Lean for Life high protein nutritional products.

■ **LEAN FOR LIFE HIGH PROTEIN NUTRITIONAL PRODUCTS :** These Drinks, Puddings, Soups, Shakes, and Pastas are a delicious, convenient way to get high biological value protein and nutrients. Over 30 different products to choose from, including a new "Variety Pack."

■ **LEAN FOR LIFE SNACK BARS:** Wildly popular with Lindora members, these bars are tasty, convenient, and satisfying. Great for sustained energy. Available in assorted flavors, including a "Variety Pack."

■ **"STARTER PACKAGES":** Everything you'll need for your Lean for Life program.

INCLUDES A 28-DAY CLINICALLY TESTED DIET PLAN THAT'S SAFE FOR TEENS!

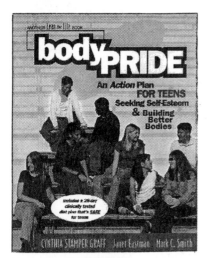

I was never an exercise person. Hated it. I'd walk down stairs and I was out of breath. Now l walk three miles a day. I get to think about everything and it gets the stress out.
—AIMEE, 16

I got it in my head that I could make the football team and I did. On the first day of tryouts, I gave more than 100 percent. I was tired but kept going, even when my friends gave up. I'm now No. 90.
—ERIC, 13

People are always talking about how kids and teens are fat, but they never tell us what to do about it...
—from the text

bodyPRIDE by Cynthia Stamper Graff, Janet Eastman and Mark C. Smith

Aimed at teens, *bodyPRIDE* emphasizes development of self-esteem as the foundation for safe, long-lasting weight loss. Written in punchy, hip prose accompanied by interactive passages and engaging illustrations, this book is highly accessible to teenagers who want to feel better about themselves so they can become motivated to set goals, eat right, exercise and lose weight.

- Contains a step-by-step program to help teens fulfill their dreams—from safely dropping 5 to 100 pounds to improving their grades, making a team, getting dates, dumping bad habits, maintaining supportive relationships and enhancing self-image.
- Based on the Lindora Medical Clinics' well-known Lean for Life® program used by thousands of adults and teens over the past 25 years.
- Includes a Daily Action Plan for measuring and celebrating progress.
- Supported by answer Hotline and World Wide Web site.
- Teaches teens to deal with pressures from friends and avoid pitfalls on and off campus.

bodyPRIDE costs $18.95 (paperback) *plus shipping and handling*

You've lost the weight. How will you keep it off?

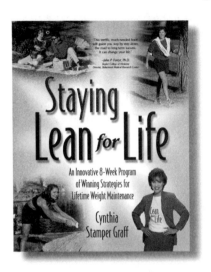

STAYING LEAN FOR LIFE by Cynthia Stamper Graff

More than 95% of people who lose weight regain it within one year. How will you make sure you're not one of them?

That's exactly what STAYING LEAN FOR LIFE is designed to help you do. Based on 27 years experience at the renowned Lindora Medical Clinics – Southern California's #1 medical weight control program – STAYING LEAN FOR LIFE guides you day-by-day through the challenges of weight maintenance. Along the way, you'll gain knowledge and develop vital, valuable skills that will help you stay focused and committed to new, healthful behaviors.

STAYING LEAN FOR LIFE is a book you live day by day. It's a book you do. Over the next eight weeks, you'll discover tried-and-true tips and strategies that will support you in making lasting changes in your life. Each day features a new topic, along with three key success strategies that are *absolutely essential* for long-term weight maintenance. You'll learn to "Eat Better", "Move More", and "Stress Less". You'll also read inspiring "Success Stories" of people who have learned what you want to know. You'll discover how to make the "Mental Fitness Circle" work for you and how your Daily Action Plan will help you stay focused and on track.

Let this proven, results-oriented program guide you step-by-step along the road to long-term success. Now that you've *lost* the weight, enjoy the experience of STAYING LEAN FOR LIFE!

"Thank you, Herman and Jean, for helping me achieve my goals. You are my 'competitive advantage', and I'm happy to share your wisdom with others." – Cynthia Graff, President, Lindora, Inc.

MENTORS™ Daily Mental Training Audio Cassette Tapes

Nationally prominent experts in the field of mental training, Herman Frankel, M.D. and Jean Staeheli work together in conducting clinical programs and research at the Portland Health Institute. They have worked with Olympic athletes, world class musicians, corporate executives, people preparing for surgery, and Lindora Medical Staff and patients. They are known for the outstanding results they help people achieve.

These tapes contain powerful tools that can assist you in making positive structural changes in your brain and your body.

BASIC PROGRAM

The audio cassette tapes in the Basic Program are the ones routinely made available to our patients and all the members of our professional staff. Each tape has the voice of Herman M. Frankel, M.D. on one side and the voice of Jean Staeheli on the other. Includes everything you need to get started in a unique program designed for results! **4 TAPES – $49.95*** *plus shipping and handling*

Tape 1	**Tape 2**	**Tape 3**	**Tape 4**
MY PEACEFUL PLACE	ENJOYING MY FOOD CHOICES	ENJOYING MY PHYSICAL ACTIVITY	RETURNING TO THE PATH
Creating your safe space; learning to rest, to focus, and to rehearse	Taking pleasures in healthy choices	Developing the habit of experiencing pleasure in your physical activity	Getting back on track, with feelings of relief, when you find you've strayed

ADVANCED TAPES

The advanced tapes deal with the most common specific issues which our staff and patients find themselves addressing as they make changes in their own lives. Like the tapes in the Basic Program, each tape has the voice of Herman M. Frankel, M.D. on one side and the voice of Jean Staeheli on the other. **$9.95* PER TAPE** *plus shipping and handling*

Tape 5	**Tape 6**	**Tape 7**	**Tape 8**	**Tape 9**
LETTING GO OF WHAT I NO LONGER NEED	THE KEEPER OF THE GARDEN OF ROSES	THE CHILD IN THE CHAMBER IN THE CASTLE	THE TRAVELER AND THE JOURNEY	MY HEALING PLACE
Becoming free from dependence on old attachments and patterns	Learning to respect boundaries and expect others to do the same	Giving and accepting nurturing, safely and genuinely	Moving beyond the familiar, accepting help, and dealing with challenges	Exploring oneself, finding sites ready for healing, and doing healing work

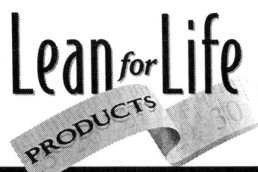

Order these great products today!

Call 1-800-LEAN 4 LI(FE)

(1-800-532-6454)

Fax 1-714-979-9752
Mail this form to: LINDORA, Inc.

3505 Cadillac Avenue, Suite N-2, Costa Mesa, CA 92626

O R D E R   F O R M

Name: _____

Address: _____

City: _____ State: _____ Zip: _____

Home Phone: _____ Work Phone: _____

PRODUCT	QUANTITY	UNIT PRICE	SUB TOTAL
LEAN FOR LIFE BOOK	_____	$18.95	$_____
MENTOR™ DAILY MENTAL TRAINING AUDIO CASSETTE TAPES (4 TAPE SET)	_____	$49.95	$_____
PEDOMETER	_____	$19.95	$_____
DR. STAMPER'S VITAMINS - #42	_____	$7.00	$_____
KETONE STRIPS - #50	_____	$12.00	$_____

Type of Payment: ☐ Discover ☐ Amex ☐ Money Order
☐ VISA ☐ MasterCard (Sorry, No Personal Checks)

Card #: _____

Exp. Date: _____

Signature: _____

SUB-TOTAL $_____

APPLICABLE SALES TAX $_____

SHIPPING COSTS $_____

TOTAL ENCLOSED $_____

HIGH PROTEIN NUTRIONAL PRODUCTS
CALL OR FAX FOR A COMPLETE LISTING OF MORE THAN 30 DELICIOUS PRODUCTS CLINICALLY PROVEN TO ENHANCE WEIGHT CONTROL RESULTS.

PLEASE COPY OR TEAR OUT TO ORDER.

ALL PRICES SUBJECT TO CHANGE WITHOUT NOTICE.